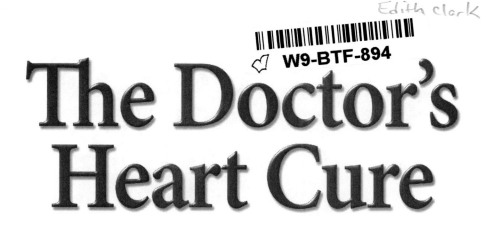

The Doctor's Heart Cure

How to Build an Impregnable Heart Today—Without Unnatural Diets, Dangerous Drugs And Time-Wasting Aerobics

Discover the simple, easy, enjoyable and above-all PROVEN plan to lose weight and achieve a shock-proof, disease-resistant heart – with delicious, natural foods and just a few minutes of exercise a day.

BY AL SEARS, M.D.

A LYNN SONBERG BOOK

The Doctor's Heart Cure

ISBN 13-digit: 978-0-938045-65-6
ISBN 10-Digit: 0-938045-65-2

Published in the United States by:
Dragon Door Publications, Inc
P.O. Box 4381, St. Paul, MN 55104
Tel: (651) 487-2180
Fax: (651) 487-3954
Credit card orders: 1-800-899-5111
Email: support@dragondoor.com
Website: www.dragondoor.com

Book design, Illustrations and cover by Derek Brigham
Website http//www.dbrigham.com
Tel/Fax: (763) 208-3069 Email: dbrigham@visi.com

Manufactured in the United States
First Edition: November 2004

DISCLAIMER
This book is is for information only. The author is not offering professional advice or services to the individual reader and the suggestions in this book are in no way a substitute for medical evaluation and recommendations by a physician. All matters concerning your health require ongoing medical supervision. Thus the author and publisher do not recommend changing your medication regimen without consulting your physician. The author and publisher are not liable or responsible for any direct loss or damage allegedly arising from any information or suggestion in this book or from the use of any treatments mentioned in this book.

The Doctor's Heart Cure
Table of Contents

Progressively challenging your heart and lungs...accelerating your heart and body's adaptation and response times...monitoring and changing exercise intensity levels...adjusting exercise duration for optimal physical development ...using your heart rate to measure intensity...target pulse ranges.

What to ask your doctor before you begin your PACE™ program...choosing the exercise activity that's best for you...sample week-by-week outline of the PACE™ plan...8-week plan at-a-glance...implementing the full tilt program...a sample, 10-minute workout plan.

Training your heart and blood vessels to deliver more oxygen faster...personalizing your plan...cycling and the risk of impotency.

The relationship between muscle size and strength...resistance training...the best exercises for functional strength... common sense calisthenics...how to strengthen your foundation by exercising your legs and lower body...strengthening your core with exercises for your abdomen and lower back...strengthening your upper body...designing your workout action plan.

How and why CoQ10 works to strengthen the heart...the remarkable benefits of CoQ10...patient evidence from the Center for Health and Wellness...the nature and functions of CoQ10.

Pumping up your mitochondria for high energy production...the Krebs cycle and ATP...the health dangers of CoQ10 deficiency...a special warning to vegans...the heart health research on CoQ10.

How CoQ10 helps lower blood pressure...reversing congestive heart failure... helps ease angina pectoris...helps you recover from heart surgery... protecting your brain with CoQ10...strengthening your immune system... recommended doses and sources for different conditions...helping with Parkinson's disease...your CoQ10 action plan.

Feeding the heart the nutrients it needs...the five most common nutrient deficiencies...why you do need supplements and what to consider...the healthy heart super-nutrients for greater protection.

L-carnitine for greater energy and fat burning capability...L-arginine for better blood circulation, a stronger heart and stronger muscles...tocopherols and tocotrienols to lower your heart risks...the many other proven health benefits of tocopherols and tocotrienols... the many benefits of Vitamin C...why you need to take extra antioxidants

More heart-smart antioxidants...ALA for energy...Carnosine as an anti-glycation agent and muscle protector...carotenoids for eyes and immunity...L-Glutamine for muscle-building growth hormone...Lutein to prevent free radical damage and protect the eyes...Lycopene to help the heart, blood vessels, and eyes...Omega-3 to prevent heart disease and cancer...Vitamin A for the eyes and as an antioxidant.

Introduction

For decades, Americans have tried to avoid heart disease by following the advice of the American Heart Association. We have strived to eat less fat, do more cardiovascular exercise, and lower our cholesterol levels. We have spent millions of dollars on low-fat foods, gym memberships, and cholesterol-lowering medications.

Despite all this effort and expense, heart disease remains both the number one disease diagnosed and the number one cause of death in the United States. Cardiovascular disease kills more than 950,000 Americans every year, according to the Centers for Disease Control and Prevention. It's hard to find an American who hasn't had a loved one disabled or killed by heart disease.

Heart disease continues as America's biggest killer for one simple reason: The health advice we try to follow is just plain wrong. Giving up meat and eggs, jogging, and taking medications *will not cure your* heart disease.

Most of us find it difficult and unpleasant to cram more "cardio" exercise into our busy schedules, to swear off the foods we love, and to count calories and grams of fat and cholesterol. The truth is that these manipulations are unnatural and unnecessary burdens that distract you from the real solution to a healthy heart. To make matters worse, following this flawed advice actually creates additional health problems.

What would you say if you learned that you could completely reverse serious heart disease in a very short period – by following advice directly opposite of the standard recommendations? In as little as a few months, the men and women in my clinic have used a few easy-to-follow steps to cure their heart disease. This book will show you the strategy for real heart health. It's time to discard the old assumptions that failed us and re-examine the facts.

A Fresh Look Leads to a Startling Conclusion

During the time when the World War II generation feasted on a breakfast of steak and eggs, obesity was relatively constant in America, hovering around 10 percent. Diabetes was relatively uncommon, with about one case of diet-related mature onset diabetes for each case of genetics-related childhood diabetes. All of this was about to change.

In 1957, the American Heart Association linked dietary fat to heart disease and recommended that Americans cut the fat in their diets. We swapped cereals for the protein-based breakfasts of our grandparents' generation, and we started struggling with low-fat diets.

Over the next couple of decades, food producers developed a wide variety of low-fat and fat-free foods. And since low-fat and fat-free foods were more profitable than natural foods, food-producing corporations were eager to promote this concept. We gobbled down these "healthy" foods, expecting to lower our risk of heart disease as we lowered our weight. But we didn't lose weight. In fact, the number of overweight Americans skyrocketed. The rate of obesity tripled, and we plunged into a new epidemic of maturity-onset diabetes.

Since following the American Heart Association's low-fat advice, the number of Americans either obese or overweight has exploded to two out of three – levels never seen anywhere in history. In 2003, the Centers for Disease Control announced that obesity will soon replace tobacco use as America's number one lifestyle-related health problem. Also during this time, the rate of maturity-onset diabetes soared. We now see nine times as many cases of diet-induced maturity-onset diabetes as we did in previous generations. This type of diabetes has also become more severe and is occurring in much younger people.

The American Heart Association's recommendations ultimately led us further away from our natural protein-based diet. And, more importantly, the low-fat approach failed in its primary goal: Heart disease continues to kill more Americans than any other disease.

Discard Failed Beliefs and Embrace Strategies That Work

Why does the conventional approach to heart disease fail? It doesn't work because it is based on *false beliefs*. To halt heart disease, you must re-think everything you've heard about this condition. This book will help you gain new wisdom about how to restore your natural heart health and avoid heart disease.

Because the old, flawed ideas continue to dominate the medical establishment, this new information may surprise you. But when you replace these failed assumptions with The *Doctor's Heart Cure's* three primary principles, you will begin to build heart health and prevent or reverse heart disease. The three key principles are:

• Dietary fat is not the culprit. **Starches – not fat – fuel heart disease.** Because low-fat diets are even higher in starches, these diets make cardiovascular disease worse.

• Long-duration cardiovascular exercise mimics prolonged stress and breaks down vital cardiopulmonary reserve. **Interval and weight training are the keys to building heart health.** "Cardio" workouts of more than about 15 minutes in duration are a waste of time and cause additional health problems.

• Cholesterol does not cause heart disease. You can monitor other factors that reveal much more about your heart health than blood cholesterol. Your cholesterol level doesn't have to stay below 200, and the drugs used to lower cholesterol are bad for your heart and your general health. Cholesterol-lowering drugs interfere with vital processes necessary for maintaining health, including energy production in your heart and your capacity to calm oxidative stress in your heart and arteries. In other words, the drugs doctors commonly prescribe to lower cholesterol do not address the true cause of heart disease – and they actually create additional problems.

The myths and misconceptions about heart disease are widespread and persistent, in part, because food processing and drug corporations capitalize on our heart disease problem. This is not to suggest some sort of secret conspiracy to keep us unhealthy. It's simply a fact that heart disease has become big business. Food manufacturers can make more profit selling a box of processed cereal than an egg, and drug companies can make more money selling new drugs than promoting exercise programs. It's time to hold these groups accountable for their products and advice. Clearly, the current approach to fighting cardiovascular disease isn't working. There must be a better way.

The effective way to beat heart disease is to root out the underlying cause. People of all ages have rebuilt youthful hearts and blood vessels. Instead of sacrifice, denial, and unwanted side effects, a natural heart health plan gives you more energy. For 16 years, patients at the Center for Health and Wellness have been feeling better, aging better, performing better, and living longer. And they achieve these goals without worry or time-consuming daily regimens. You can share their improved health, and you can do so without eating foods you don't like or becoming a vegetarian. My program includes no confusing double-talk, no burdensome counting of calories or fat grams, and no toxic drugs.

Re-thinking Heart Disease: A New Model for Heart Health

The Doctor's Heart Cure creates a new paradigm for healing heart disease and achieving heart health. This book provides a detailed program that flies in the face of conventional guidelines. Extensive scientific research and experience with thousands of patients supports this approach. My patients have improved their cardiac health and overall physical condition by using these strategies, which have been proven to work.

In addition, *The Doctor's Heart Cure* Program is much easier to follow than the American Heart Association guidelines. We have an instinctive desire for foods that are naturally fatty, salty, or sweet. With a few adaptations to our modern world, these natural preferences can serve you well. The low-fat diet is unnatural, and the chronic denial of enjoyable food is unnecessary. The key to heart-healthy eating is to choose natural, unprocessed foods that you like.

Similarly, few people enjoy pounding away on a treadmill for thirty minutes to an hour at a time. Many people who try to stick to this time-consuming exercise routine find that their instincts cry out for them to stop. Those people who endure extended cardio workouts unwittingly produce unwanted changes in their bodies such as the loss of muscle, bone density, and internal organ weight. In addition, they often wind up with overuse injuries. Patients don't complain when they discover that the core of *The Doctor's Heart Cure's* exercise program is workouts that last no more than 20 minutes and can be completed in as little as six minutes.

Lastly, the popular strategy of monitoring cholesterol is ineffective, and the prescribed medications are toxic. Most patients who use cholesterol-lowering drugs don't know that the medications are making them weak and tired and causing their muscles to ache if they try to exercise. My patients are delighted to enjoy increased energy and well-being when they switch to effective natural alternatives to these medications.

In addition, compelling evidence indicates that the best blood predictor of heart disease risk is not cholesterol but homocysteine. This turns out to be great news: It's much easier and less toxic to your body to lower homocysteine levels than to lower cholesterol levels.

COMMUNICATE WITH YOUR DOCTOR

It's important to have a doctor you feel comfortable with to help you make effective decisions about your health. Use the information in this book to talk about your options to strengthen your heart. Advise your physician about any herbs, nutritional supplements, or other over-the-counter products you plan to take. Some of these natural remedies can interfere with test results or cause unwanted effects.

It's important to let your physician know about the steps you are taking to combat cardiovascular disease and improve your health. The best way to help your doctor help you is to work with him or her to develop a program that will best suit your individual needs.

Using This Book: A Stepwise Process

The Doctor's Heart Cure leads you through a two-step process to build heart health. In Step One, "How Modern Medicine Missed the Boat," you'll come to understand why researchers and physicians went astray in their approach to heart disease.

- Chapter 1 lets you know how the ever-increasing adulteration of our food supply made the problems with cardiovascular health progressively worse over the years. The problem began with the evolution of agriculture and food technology. The problem turned into a crisis in the last generation when the so-called "heart healthy diet" the American Heart Association advocated became popular. This program is *unhealthy*, and it makes heart disease worse.
- Chapter 2 examines how long-duration cardiovascular exercise for heart disease robs your heart and lungs of capacity, zaps your body of strength and muscle, and accelerates several unhealthy aspects of aging.
- Chapter 3 tells why cholesterol testing is all wrong, and what markers doctors should be checking.
- Chapter 4 gives you the lowdown on the far too-commonly used dangerous heart drugs and their harmful side effects. It describes how cholesterol-lowering drugs deplete energy reserves, lower sexual vigor, and interfere with one of your cardiovascular system's most important antioxidant systems. It explains that blood pressure medications can de-condition your heart and interfere with effective exercise, and that the overuse of medications for heart disease can cause serious health problems.

- **Chapter 5** advises you about effective screening tests – which most doctors don't do – to assess heart health. Tests for five indicators in the blood – levels of coenzyme Q10, homocysteine, C-reactive protein, insulin, and essential fats – reveal an abundance of useful information about heart health. You'll also find some measures you can do yourself.

Step Two is "Your Action Plan for Heart Health" to prevent or reverse heart disease.

- In chapter 6, you can learn about a surprising plan for eating and enjoying real food, including good fats, protein, and plenty of fruits and vegetables. This plan deviates in important ways from both the American Heart Association's low-fat recommendations and the Atkins-like low-carbohydrate group of diets. You will discover how to emulate the eating patterns of our past, before heart disease was an epidemic. This means looking beyond counting either fat or carbs to finding the quality of fat, protein, and carbohydrate that nature provided us for eons.
- In chapter 7, you'll discover the secret of how you can exercise less and get better results! You can follow the 8-week program of progressive activity that takes less time and is more effective than traditional cardiovascular workouts. You will improve your cardiac, pulmonary, and blood vessel response to exertion. Not only will this program improve your cardiovascular health, it also will transform your body, as you burn fat and build muscle and strength.
- One nutrient, *coenzyme Q10,* is so important that it merits a chapter of its own. Find out how to use it to energize your heart in Chapter 8.
- By the time you complete chapter 9, you'll know how to supplement your diet with four additional nutrients every heart needs – although most people don't consume them in sufficient quantities. L-carnitine, L-arginine, tocopherols, and vitamin C are essential for a healthy heart. You will see why these supplements are important, how to get them, and how much to take.
- In chapter 10 you will learn how to reduce inflammation and control

oxidation of blood vessels. This key component of your heart-healthy program tells you how you can use antioxidants to reduce oxidative stress, and about the role of B vitamins in reducing homocysteine levels.

- If you suffer from high blood pressure, diabetes, loss of muscle, or obesity – problems that often accompany cardiovascular disease – you can customize your own program using chapter 11 to guide you.
- The final chapter helps you put it all together with an action plan of how to implement your *Doctor's Heart Cure* for life.

STEP ONE

How Mainstream Medicine Missed the Boat

1

Modern Nutrition
and the Diet Disaster

Mankind created the modern epidemic of heart disease. Over millions of years, our hearts have evolved and adapted to our natural environment. In recent history, however, we have radically changed the way we treat our hearts. When you look at the big picture, it comes as no coincidence that heart disease first appeared about 10,000 years ago, the same time our ancestors discovered agriculture.

Simply put, in the millions of years before agriculture, we ate foods high in protein and fat and low in carbohydrates. In the few thousand years since, we switched to a diet high in carbohydrates and low in fat and protein. With this change came the beginning of heart disease.

To prevent and reverse heart disease, you must change your Western diet to follow more closely the eating patterns of your hunter-gatherer ancestors, who relied on foods that grew naturally in their environment. If you eat the foods you are genetically designed to handle, you can avoid almost all of the heart disease that threatens you today.

As you will see in this chapter, it is possible to rediscover your natural diet. You can look at the archaeological record of our prehistoric ancestors and the remarkable health of surviving pre-agrarian people. You can track the health consequences that follow a shift to a grain-based diet, as well as the changes that followed the adoption of the medical establishment's "heart healthy" diet in our lifetime.

If you want to get right to the action plan for returning to eating your natural diet in a modern world, you can skip ahead to Chapter 6. You will find this change in diet surprisingly easy. As you will see, eating naturally doesn't rely on denial or strength of will because you retain the instinctive tastes of your Paleolithic hunter-gatherer relatives.

Avoid the Nutritional Disaster of the Agrarian Society

We may be better dressed and live in more comfortable houses than our prehistoric relatives, but human beings really haven't changed much in the past 400,000 years. In fact, our genes are 99.99 percent identical to those of our ancient ancestors. If you met one of your pre-agrarian relatives on the street today, you wouldn't be able to spot him in a crowd.

But what did our ancestors really eat? We can learn about the lifestyles our relatives had before agriculture by studying the fossil record and by researching modern hunter-gatherer societies. Studies of modern hunter-gatherer societies show that all derive more than half of their subsistence from animal foods.[1]

Nutritionists may cringe at the thought of such dependence on animal foods, but if you compare the modern diet and the hunter-gatherer diet, you'll uncover some startling facts. These hunter-gatherer relatives thrived on a diet of lean game meat, supplemented with some vegetables, occasional nuts and seeds, and seasonal fresh fruits and berries, when available. Those who lived near water ate fish and seafood. Eggs were a special treat. Contrary to popular opinion, our ancestors were more hunter than gatherer. Research shows that their diets averaged 65 percent energy from meat and fat and only 35 percent from plant sources.

At the time, humans rarely if ever ate cereal grains. Grains are virtually indigestible by the human digestive tract unless the grains are milled and cooked. Grinding stones don't appear in the fossil record until 10,000 to 15,000 years ago, the time of the Agricultural Revolution.

You No Longer Have to Trade Quality for Quantity

The introduction of agriculture marked a significant change in the way we ate. The switch to farming could support a much larger population, but it also created a problem: We traded food quality for quantity, but our genes remain essentially unchanged. A few thousand years isn't enough time for our bodies to genetically adapt to these new foods. We are genetically equipped to consume the high-protein, low-carbohydrate diet our hunter-gather ancestors ate, but our diets shifted to a high-carbohydrate, low-protein diet common in agricultural societies.

The effect on human health was immediate and profound. Paleo-anthropologists found that whenever grains became the staple in human diets, there was a universal drop in height, muscularity, and brain size. Archaeologists can easily tell if newly discovered bones are from a hunter-gatherer society or an agricultural one. The hunter-gatherers are taller, have stronger and thicker bones, much better teeth, and are more robust than their agricultural descendants. The remains of people from agricultural societies have decayed teeth, fragile bones, and signs of chronic disease.

When man switched to a grain-based diet, we became physically shorter. Fossil evidence shows that European big-game hunters of 30,000 years ago were an average of six inches taller than their farmer descendants. One of these most striking examples occurs in Greece. Studies have found that the average hunter-gatherer in Greece was 5 foot 9 inches tall, while the average height of these same people shrank to just 5 feet when they became farmers. Despite all the modern advances in public health, the modern day Greek has still not recovered the height of their pre-agrarian ancestors.

The archeological record also shows that the epidemic of modern chronic diseases appeared at the same time we switched to a diet based on agriculture. Consider the fossils found at the burial mounds of native people in the Illinois and Ohio River valleys. Archaeologists excavated 800 skeletons that show that when these people switched from a hunter-gatherer culture to one dependent on maize farming, they experienced a 50 percent increase in malnutrition, a four-fold increase in iron-deficiency anemia, and a three-fold increase in infectious disease compared to their hunter-gatherer ancestors.[1]

Anthropologists who study indigenous cultures, some of which survived unaffected by the modern world into the 21st century, also support this link between diet and disease. We find that modern people who eat the traditional hunter-gatherer diet are astonishingly free of modern disease! In many cases, we can compare primitive people eating a hunter-gatherer diet with those of their modernized relatives who live in nearby communities and eat a grain-based diet. We don't find heart disease, cancer, diabetes, arthritis, or other diseases of civilization among the primitives. On the other hand, their modernized kinsmen who eat grains and processed foods develop all of these life-threatening conditions.

One researcher – Dr. Weston Price – traveled throughout the world and documented the lifestyles of 14 remaining hunter-gatherer cultures[2]. He discovered two features common to every one of these primitive cultures: they all lacked modern heart disease, and they all ate meat. There was not a single vegetarian in the group.

We Are All Descendants of Hunter-Gatherers

Dr. Loren Cordain, an expert on primitive dietary habits and a professor of exercise physiology at Colorado State University, examined the diets of 229 of the world's remaining native societies. He, too, found no vegetarian cultures. In fact, game was their principal source of protein and fat. Interestingly, they often reserved the organ meat for the most privileged. This preference for organ meat has important nutritional implications for heart health we will examine later. The fact that native pre-agricultural societies universally ate more protein than the average modern diet surprises many people who've heard that we eat too much protein.

Protein, Carbohydrates, and Fat in American versus Pre-Agrarian Diet

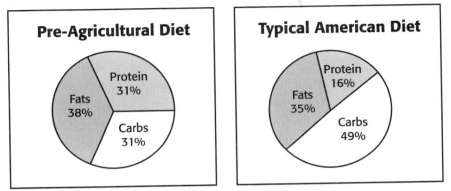

Information from The Paleo Diet (2002) by L. Cordain[3]

As you can see from the graph, we actually eat much less protein than our ancestors did! We also eat less fat and more carbohydrates than the historical norm.

We can no longer deny the evidence. Human cultures were never vegetarians. Quite the opposite: for millions of years, *we ate meat*. In fact, the more meat a society eats, the healthier it appears to be. For instance, the Masai of east Africa – who live on raw milk, cattle blood, organs, and meat – have virtually no heart disease. And the Dinkas, people who live along the banks of the Nile River and live mostly on fish and shellfish, live with no apparent heart disease, obesity, or cancer, according to a Western physician who lived among them for 15 years[4].

Dump the High-Starch, Low-Fat Diet Now

Over the past 100 years or so, food manufacturers developed new ways of milling flour that strips the wheat germ from the grain, to make refined white flour. This product is far less perishable, making it a boon to food manufacturers that want their products to last as long as possible.

Today, refined flour has become a staple in foods. But, once again, food manufacturers have traded quality nutrition for quantity and convenience.

Refined grain has been stripped of its vitamin E and several other nutrients, including the B vitamins and several minerals. Since refining grain, food manufacturers have created foods that have become increasingly less natural. We shifted from a dependence on natural carbohydrates to highly processed carbohydrates.

We could have learned from our Paleolithic ancestors. Our bodies are ill equipped to handle processed carbohydrates. Not surprisingly, we saw a dramatic rise in heart attacks and other health problems in the second half of the twentieth century when we began eating these refined foods.

Scientists noted the health epidemic, but they misdiagnosed the cause. Without a thorough understanding of the evidence, scientists identified fat as the culprit in causing heart disease.

How did such a *big fat lie* become widely accepted as fact? In part, epidemiologists saw higher rates of heart disease in the developed West than in Third World countries, and they looked for dietary factors to explain the change. They noted that Americans ate more meat and fat than poorer countries with lower rates of heart disease. Therefore, they wrongly concluded, animal fat must cause heart disease. This assumption seemed reasonable, but new evidence from other cultures caused some researchers to reconsider.

Why didn't artic Native Americans – with their very-high-fat diet of red meat and seal and whale blubber – get heart disease? What about the French who eat more fat than Americans, yet have lower heart disease rates? Scientists at first dismissed these and other exceptions as curious paradoxes. It wasn't until the hunter-gatherer researchers compiled their data that the error became obvious.

In previous studies, we thought we compared our agrarian diet with the original diet of Third World farmers. In fact, we compared our agrarian diet with their agrarian diet. The truth is the agrarian diet has not long been the natural diet of any of the people on Earth. The diet of Third World farmers already changed at the time of agrarian development.

Their diet was high in starches and low in protein and fat. Although heart disease also exists in the Third World, it is not severe when farmers use their own physical labor to farm their own local crops. It is also partially masked by the short life spans and huge infectious disease problem in these poor farmer cultures. The majority didn't live long enough to suffer from heart attacks but heart disease had already begun.

Going Back to Our Roots

The real solution to our dietary woes would require a return to our hunter diet, but this was not popular in the 1970s. Instead, we blamed eating meat for our health problems in response to the cultural and political mood of the time.

The federal government officially endorsed the blame-the-fat philosophy in 1977. A Senate Committee George McGovern led released "Dietary Goals for the United States." The publication told Americans to drastically cut their dietary fat intake, blaming dietary fat for the epidemic of the heart disease sweeping the nation. The National Institutes of Health jumped on the "ban the fat" wagon. In 1984, they announced that Americans must cut their fat intake. The American Heart Association and the media then joined in, believing that the secret to heart health is eating a low-fat diet.

Stop Starches From Ruining Your Health

The food industry produced a wide range of "low-fat" products, but without the tasty fat, the food was bland. The manufacturers solved that problem by adding sugar. In the end, we replaced dietary fat with refined carbohydrates and massive amounts of sugar in our diets. The amount of calories from fat in our American diet decreased, and the amount of calories from refined carbohydrates increased – dramatically.

This low-fat solution set the stage for a modern dietary disaster. We found out one thing for sure: if we eat excessive amounts of carbohydrates, we're going to get fat. That's why obesity levels have skyrocketed. In fact, rates of obesity were constant at about 13 percent through the 1960s and 1970s, then they suddenly began a dramatic rise. Obesity[4] is now at an astounding 25 percent! These rates began rising at the time the health authorities told us to eat low-fat.

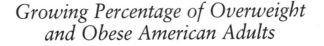

Growing Percentage of Overweight and Obese American Adults

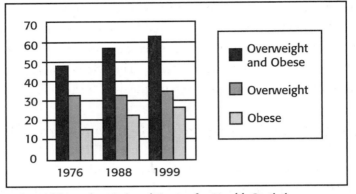

Adapted from the National Center for Health Statistics

We could have predicted this would happen. If we set aside the lifetime of prejudice against fat, we can understand the science. The hormone insulin controls fat production and in particular triggers the formation of abdominal fat. The body secretes insulin when we consume carbohydrates. The more carbohydrates you eat, the more insulin you secrete and the more fat you form, all other things being equal. Fat in the diet, in contrast, is *neutral*, in that it has little or no effect on insulin secretion.

The high insulin levels brought on from excessive carbohydrate intake affects body fat in two main ways. First, it tells your body to divert the energy from the food you eat into body fat. Second, it prevents your body from burning stored body fat for energy.[5] Ultimately, high levels of insulin make you fat and tired.

Avoid AGEs and Prevent Cardiovascular Aging

We recently learned of a new mechanism that explains how carbohydrates and processed starches directly cause heart disease. People who eat too many refined carbohydrates have sugar that sticks to the protein of their cells, damaging the protein and creating Advanced Glycation End-products (AGEs). AGEs accelerate the aging of the cardiovascular system. People with blocked arteries tend to have the highest levels of AGEs.

To make matters worse, eating carbohydrates makes you crave more carbohydrates. When you eat carbohydrates, your high insulin level triggers your hypothalamus – the part of your brain that regulates hormones – to send out hunger signals that cause you to crave even more carbohydrates. This prompts you to eat more and keeps this vicious cycle going. To interrupt this pattern, you need to do something different – *you need to eat fat and keep your carbohydrate intake low.* This allows you to lose body fat and helps to control carbohydrate cravings.

Lower Your Carbohydrate Intake to Lose Weight

It comes as no surprise that studies have found low-fat diets are disastrous for your health and ineffective for weight loss. A University of Cincinnati study concluded that patients on a very-low-carbohydrate diet lost significantly more weight than those on a low-fat, low-calorie diet in a six-month period. Even more importantly, the low carbohydrate group also lost more body fat than the low-fat group.[6]

Another study that examined people eating very-low-fat diets (14 percent fat) concluded that there was no improvement in body composition, blood sugar levels, insulin levels, or blood pressure levels. The study's authors called very low-fat diets "counterproductive" to health. [7]

Keep Your Calcium and More Vital Nutrients

There are other problems emerging from the low-fat advice. The lower fat intake itself can be detrimental to your health. One study published in the *American Journal of Clinical Nutrition* found that low-fat diets affect calcium absorption. The study found low-fat diets were associated with 20 percent lower calcium absorption than higher fat diets.[8] The State University of New York at Buffalo also found that people who eat low-fat diets develop weaker immune systems.[9] A certain amount of fat is necessary for the body to absorb vitamins. Your body cannot absorb the fat-soluble nutrients like vitamins A, D, E, and K and coenzyme CoQ10 without fat.

Maintain Vigorous Vital Organs

Here's another problem: When you eat a low-fat diet, you not only eat more carbohydrates but you also inadvertently sacrifice the most important nutrient, protein. If you follow the flawed low-fat advice, you will lose vital muscle – including heart muscle – and burden your heart with flab.

A growing number of studies back these claims, but governmental organizations stubbornly cling to their low-fat beliefs. Conventional medicine does not accept new nutritional solutions readily, if at all, no matter how useful they may be. Traditional medicine censored innovations like eating limes to ward off scurvy for up to 50 years before successfully using this new knowledge. Plus, given the information overload physicians must keep up with today, many are simply misinformed about what constitutes a healthy diet. Unfortunately, too many uninformed doctors make recommendations that make their patients' health problems worse. Eating a low-fat, high-carbohydrate diet not only makes you fatter, but it also puts you at risk for a slew of medical problems, from the onset of diabetes to heart disease and stroke.

Did Dr. Atkins Get It Right?

A generation ago, Dr. Robert Atkins changed the world of nutrition with a radical weight-loss diet that dared to confront conventional nutrition. He claimed that the best way to lose weight was not to follow a low-fat diet but a low-carbohydrate diet.

Many people severely criticized Dr. Atkins even after his death. They called him "Dr. Fatkins," and released his medical records indicating that at the time of his death, he weighed 258 pounds, a weight that would have classified him as obese.

This is unfair and incorrect. I actually met Dr. Atkins, and he appeared in good health several days before he slipped on the ice and fell into a fatal coma. He was not fat and appeared in remarkably good condition for his 72 years. Physicians gave Dr. Atkins steroids to control the swelling that developed after his head trauma. This medication caused the bloating and weight gain he experienced in his final days.

Recent studies show that Dr. Atkins's low-carbohydrate approach was on to something:

- **February 2003:** A landmark study compared the American Heart Association's low-fat diet to the Atkins' low-carbohydrate diet. The Atkins' diet caused greater weight loss and lowered cholesterol and triglycerides much more effectively than a low-fat diet of equal calories.
- **May 2003:** The prestigious *New England Journal of Medicine* published a study that found the Atkins approach beat out the American Heart Association's low-fat approach for both weight loss and blood fat improvement.
- **Nutrition Week 2003:** Preliminary results of a study the Heritage Medical Center performed on patients with Metabolic Syndrome showed heart healthy changes with a low-carb diet. (Metabolic Syndrome is a diet-induced disease causing cholesterol problems, obesity, lack of energy, high blood pressure, heart disease, and diabetes.) Participants ate a low-carbohydrate diet for 18 months. This reduced their LDL (bad) cholesterol by an average of 82 percent, and increased HDL (good) cholesterol scores by an average of 30 percent.

So, should you switch to a diet of bacon, hot dogs, and butter? No. Although you may lose weight on such a high-fat diet because it is low in carbohydrates, this diet would not make you healthy. Dr. Atkins accurately diagnosed the cause of the modern epidemics of obesity, diabetes, and heart disease, but he prescribed the wrong solution.

Refine the Atkins Approach and Get Rid of Bad Fats

It's true that fat does not have a significant effect on the hormones affecting your metabolism, but there are compelling reasons for you to avoid typical Western fat. The animal husbandry industry is responsible for unnatural living conditions of the animals that adulterate the fat. They prevent animals from getting exercise, and they feed the animals a diet of grains instead of grasses, creating obese, diseased animals.

The wild grazing animals that formed the centerpiece of the hunter-gatherer diet contained only 2 or 3 percent fat. Today's beef cattle are from 25 to 50 percent fat or more.[10] Segments of the animal husbandry industry inject domestic animals with antibiotics, hormones, and other drugs to make them market-ready in record time. This mechanization of animal husbandry produces huge corporate profits as well as a public health disaster.

Too many Atkins dieters fill their plates with *poor quality fats*. All of the herbicides, pesticides, toxins, and hormones that the animal has been exposed to collect in the fat. When you eat this animal fat, you are eating from the cesspool of toxins that have collected in the animal.

In addition, the vegetable fat that you get in the modern Western diet is an abomination. It does not resemble fat in our natural environment. Manufacturers process vegetable fats to extend their shelf life. The process creates unhealthy hydrogenation and cancer-causing trans-fatty acids. The number one fat used in food processing is corn oil, perhaps the unhealthiest fat of all.

The Atkins approach came close to nailing the problem. But just as it ignored the problem of adulterated animal fat in the modern mechanized animal industry, it fails to recognize that farming and refining changed the quality of our carbohydrate as well as its quantity.

If you want to live a long and healthy life, eat like your pre-agrarian ancestors did. To do this we must look beyond the counting grams of fat the AHA recommends or the counting grams of carbohydrate that has become so popular. We must return to the balance of high protein and fat and low-carbohydrate and we must restore the quality of these nutrients we have lost.

You can reap the biggest health changes fastest by switching to a diet high in good-quality protein. The Greeks knew protein was the most important food when they named it: 'pro-' means first, primary, of most importance, and '-tein' means food. In chapter 6, you can target healthy sources of the highest quality protein for your diet.

Reap Hunter-Gatherer Benefits Now!

While we may not want to go back into the cave, there's no reason we can't eat our easy, pre-agrarian diet. Hundreds of patients have transformed their bodies and their health – from fat and sickly to lean and vigorous. The Center for Health and Wellness is filled with patients who used to take multiple medications for heart disease, and now they take none. They grew lean, improved their cholesterol profiles, lowered their triglyceride levels, resolved their high blood pressure, and reversed their diabetes – and you can, too. Returning to eating your truly natural diet is one of the most important steps you can take to strengthen your heart and improve your overall health.

The good news is that following a natural diet isn't as hard as you may think. You can recover from the harmful effects caused by farming, weak science, and bad advice sooner than you may consider possible. You will be eating better tasting foods, you will feel more satisfied, and you will begin building heart health and reversing heart disease now.

Footnotes Chapter 1

1 Cordain L, Miller JB, Eaton SB, et al. Plant-animal subsistence ratios and macronutrient energy estimations in worldwide hunter-gatherer diets. *The American Journal of Clinical Nutrition.* 2000 Mar; 71(3);682-692.

2 Price WA. Nutrition and physical degeneration. A comparison of primitive and modern diets and their effects. NY: P.B. Hoeber, 1939.

3 Cordain L. *The Paleo Diet: Lose Weight and Get Healthy By Eating the Food You Were Designed to Eat.* NY: Wiley & Sons, 2002.

4 Obesity is defined as a Body Mass Index score of 25 or higher. The BMI is an index of acceptable weight ranges frequently used by the American Medical Association. It gauges your weight according to your height and gender. If you're 25 percent above the standard figure, you are defined as overweight. If you're 50 percent above it, you're classified as obese.

5 Morgenthaler J and Simms M. *The Low-Carb Anti-Aging Diet: Slow Aging and Lose Weight.* Smart Publications, 2000; p. 15.

6 Brehm BJ, Seeley RJ, Daniels SR and D'Allessio DA. A randomized trial comparing a very low carbohydrate diet and a calorie restricted low-fat diet on bodyweight and cardiovascular risk factors in healthy women. *Journal of Clinical Endocrine Metabolism.* 2003 Apr; 88(4):1617-1623.

7 Knopp RH, Walden CE, Retzlaff BM, et al. Long-term cholesterol-lowering effects of 4 fat-restricted diets in hypercholesterolemic and combined hyperlipidemic men. The Dietary Alternatives Study. *Journal of the American Medical Association.* 1997 Nov 12; 278(18):1509-1515.

8 Wolf RL, Cauley JA, Baker CE, et al. Factors associated with calcium absorption efficiency in pre- and perimenopausal women. *American Journal of Clinical Nutrition,* 2000 Aug; 72(2):466-471.

9 Venkatraman JT, Leddy J, and Pendergast D. Dietary fats and immune status in athletes: clinical implications. *Medicine Science of Sports Exercise,* 2000 Jul; 32(7Suppl):S389-95.

10 Schmid RF. *Traditional Foods Are Your Best Medicine.* Healing Arts Press, Rochester, Vermont, 1997; p. 51.

2

Sidestep the "Cardio" Exercise Myth

Pick up almost any book or magazine on exercise and you'll probably read the standard exercise prescription: For cardiovascular health, work out for 30 to 60 minutes three or four times a week. You may have heard the same advice from your physician. There's one simple problem with this generic exercise prescription: It doesn't work.

In fact, long-duration exercise is a waste of your time, and can actually cause other health problems. This type of exercise makes the heart and lungs more efficient, but it *reduces their reserve capacity*. Simply put, your reserve capacity is your body's ability to respond effectively to sudden demands you place on it. For your heart, reserve capacity is crucial. It can mean the difference between a long healthy life and sudden death from a heart attack.

When you exercise continuously for more than about 10 minutes, your heart adapts by becoming more efficient. It achieves this efficiency through downsizing. Long-duration exercise makes the heart, lungs, and muscles smaller so that they can go longer with less energy, but there's a trade-off. The cardiovascular system becomes very good at handling a 60-minute jog, but it *gives up* the ability to provide you with big bursts of energy for short periods. Far from protecting your heart, this loss makes you more vulnerable to a heart attack.

You can strengthen your heart and build reserve capacity by following a specific program I have developed during years of working with athletes, trainers, and patients at the Center for Health and Wellness. This program is called PACE™ or Progressively Accelerating Cardiopulmonary Exertion™. You can forget about working for hours at the gym! You can build a strong heart to handle your life's demands more effectively with the PACE™ system. This simple-to-follow system takes only about *10 minutes* a day!

Now if you're chomping at the bit to get started with your PACE™ program, you can jump directly to Chapter 7, Build a Strong Heart: Get More for Less. To get a firm foundation of the theory behind my exercise program, just keep reading. You'll see why the PACE™ program works – and why the standard cardiovascular exercise recommendation is the wrong kind of exercise for your heart. This information can help motivate you and keep the skeptics at bay.

Train your Heart with Intervals, Not Endurance Exercise

Conventional wisdom holds that your heart needs endurance training for optimal health. In fact, in November 2002, the federal government's Institute of Medicine issued the recommendation that Americans strive to exercise at least one hour per day.

Heart attacks don't happen due to a lack of endurance. They typically come about when a person is either at rest or when there's a sudden, sizable demand on the heart. Heart attacks often strike when someone lifts a heavy object, has sex, or experiences an unexpected emotional blow. For one reason or another, the oxygen supply to the heart can't keep up with a change in demand.

The right kind of exercise builds the heart's ability to respond effectively to these demands. You can indeed increase both your heart's maximal capacity and its speed at increasing its output to respond to demand. Yet long-duration exercise does not help you do this. In fact, it has the *opposite* effect by forcing the heart to become smaller and more efficient. The body trades the ability to handle big demands for the ability to go farther.

Studies have demonstrated that short-duration exercise improves cardiovascular health more than long-duration exercise. A recent Harvard study found that men who performed shorter bouts of exercise reduced their heart disease risk by 20 percent.[1] In other words, the men who did high-intensity, interval exercise reduced their heart disease risk by 100 percent more than those who did endurance exercise.

Dr. Stephen Seiler recently compared 20 minutes of running on a treadmill to running for 2 minutes followed by 2 minutes of rest for five cycles. He reported at the American College of Sports Medicine that interval exercise improved maximal cardiac outputs while continuous exercise did not. Intervals also produced another important improvement not seen with continuous exercise, the development of quicker cardiac adjustments to changes in demand. The interval trainees also achieved "higher peak stroke volumes." Think of peak stroke volume as the horsepower of your heart. It is the highest volume of blood your heart can pump per beat when challenged.

Interval training also lowers cholesterol levels. And, more importantly, it can improve your cholesterol ratios. Patients at the Center for Health and Wellness and a recent study conducted in Ireland confirm this finding. Researchers studied middle-aged, sedentary men and women who performed ten-minute bouts of exercise throughout the day for six weeks. The blood tests of the men and women showed both a drop in total cholesterol and a rise in beneficial HDL cholesterol.[2]

Interval training also helps exercisers maintain healthy testosterone levels. A study in the *Journal of Applied Physiology* found that testosterone levels increase more in men who do interval exercise than in those doing endurance training. Interestingly, the oldest men in the study obtained the most dramatic results.[3] This is good news because more youthful testosterone levels help older men maintain their muscle mass, libido, and bone integrity.

Now let's look at the physical effects of long-duration exercise by considering the extreme example of continuous-duration conditioned athletes such as long-distance runners. The marathon originated with the professional Athenian distance runner, Pheidippides, in 490 B.C. He achieved fame by running 26.2 miles from Marathon to Athens. He announced the victory of the Greeks over the Persian navy at Marathon, then "collapsed of exhaustion and died."

Also consider the story of marathoner, Jim Fixx, who preached that long-duration cardiovascular endurance training was the best method for achieving optimal health. He practiced what he preached, right up to the moment he dropped dead of a heart attack – while running.

Every year very well-conditioned long-distance runners suffer sudden cardiac death. Distance runners have higher rates of sudden cardiac death than other athletes do. Modern marathons have emergency stations specifically equipped to handle the abnormal heart rhythms, heart attacks, and other cardiac emergencies that can be expected to occur. This increased risk appears regardless of culture or diet.

Long-distance running has a detrimental effect on the health of your blood fats. Scientists in Barcelona, Spain, examined the blood of long-distance runners and found that after a workout they experienced an increase in both the blood levels of and the oxidation of LDL cholesterol and triglycerides.[4]

Worse yet, a report in the *American Journal of Cardiology* found that distance running disrupted the balance of blood thinners and thickeners, elevating clotting levels and inflammatory factors.[5] These changes are signs of heart distress, not a heart that's becoming stronger after exercise.

The bottom line is that to use your willpower to force yourself into frequently repeating continuous "cardio" is not mimicking the natural condition. In nature, our path, pace, stride, intensity, positioning, and force during exercise all occur in starts and stops to meet the changing demands of our surroundings. Your body is designed to work in interval bursts.

For heart health, forget about endurance exercise. Brief intervals of exercise build a stronger heart and circulatory system to handle your real life demands more effectively than long-duration exercise.

Shed More Fat with Interval Exercise

Most people think that the longer they work out, the more weight they will lose. They plod on mile after sweaty mile, assuming that they are melting off unwanted fat with every step. In fact, these dedicated but misinformed exercisers are undermining their own efforts! Endurance exercise is not the best way to lose body fat. *Long-term exercise calls on the body to store more fat!*

While this may be contrary to much of what you've heard about exercise, the following chart helps us understand how this misconception became so widespread.

Nutrient	At Rest	Low Intensity	Moderate Intensity	High Intensity
Protein	1-5%	5-8%	2-5%	2%
Carbs	35%	70%	40%	95%
Fat	60%	15%	55%	3%

SOURCE: *Revisiting Energy Systems, May 2002, IDEA Health and Fitness Source, adapted from McArdle W.D., et.al. 1999. Sports & Exercise Nutrition. New York: Lippincott Williams & Wilkins.*

By studying the chart, you see that the body burns the greatest amount of fat (55 percent) during moderate-intensity exercise. This led many people to the false conclusion that you burn the greatest amount of fat by long, moderate-intensity exercise. While this is true during the 30 or 60 minutes you are working out, it does not take into account the changes in your metabolism after you stop exercising.

Your body is always adapting to the demands put on it. When you burn fat during exercise, you are telling your body to maintain fat stores so that they will be available for the next exercise session. In essence, your body hoards your fat reserves to use as fuel for future workouts. Instead of decreasing fat, this type of endurance exercise triggers your body to make more fat whenever possible. Now if you look back at the graph, you'll see that you get the highest percentage of your energy needs from fat while you are at rest. But you wouldn't use this strategy to burn fat! That fact seems to have gone unnoticed.

Endurance exercise actually *encourages* fat production. When you begin working out, your body burns ATP, the highest energy fuel in the body, but there is only enough ATP for one or two minutes of exercise. Next, your body switches to glycogen, a carbohydrate stored in muscle tissue. Your glycogen stores will take you through about 15 minutes of exercise. After that, your body taps into its fat reserves for fuel.

This fat-burning strategy may at first sound like an ideal approach to exercise for weight loss, but it isn't. Since your body does all it can to adapt to demands, it builds back your fat the next time you eat to prepare you for the next time you exercise for a long time. It also sacrifices other tissues, such as muscle, to preserve fat whenever possible.

One of the primary reasons people choose the wrong form of exercise is that they presume that their body changes during an exercise session. It never does. All the important changes begin *after you stop* working out. They are consequences of your body adapting to prepare for the next time you ask your body to perform that same activity.

This happens with many patients at the Center for Health and Wellness. A number of studies also confirm the phenomenon. For example, researchers at Colorado State University measured how long our bodies continue to burn fat after brief periods of exercise. Study participants exercised for 20 minutes in sets of two-minute intervals of exercise, and one-minute rest periods. The researchers found that participants still burned fat 16 hours after the interval exercising! At rest, their fat oxidation was up by 62 percent, and their resting metabolic rate rose 4 percent.[6] In other words, interval exercise continues to trigger fat burning long after the session is over.

During brief sessions of interval training, the body burns the energy stored in the muscle tissue, rather than energy stored in fat. Over time, this teaches your body to store more energy in the muscles – not as fat – so that it will be available for quick bursts of energy. You also teach your body that storing energy as fat is inefficient because you never exercise long enough to use fat as your primary fuel source.

Other studies demonstrate the effectiveness of short, high-intensity interval exercise at burning body fat. In one study, researchers at Laval University in Quebec compared long, moderate-intensity, aerobic exercise with high-intensity short interval exercise. There were two study groups: a long-duration group that cycled for 45 minutes without stopping, and a short-interval exercise group that cycled in numerous short bouts (lasting from 15 to 90 seconds), with rests between intervals. The long-duration group burned twice as many calories as the interval group, but the short-interval group lost more fat. In fact, for every calorie burned, the interval group lost *nine* times more fat.[7]

Another benefit to the high-intensity interval approach is that it doesn't take as long. The PACE™ program takes *less than 15 minutes a day*. A Stanford University School of Medicine study demonstrated that just ten intense minutes of exercise helps you lose body fat – and that can fit into almost any schedule.[8]

> ♥ *Exercising in short bursts helps you lose weight. You burn carbohydrates stored in your muscles during exercise, then you burn fat after you stop exercising.*

Begin PACE™ Now to Live Longer

Low-intensity exercise is also not the most effective way of living longer. A study in May 2003 of almost 2,000 British men looked at the relationship between death and low-level endurance. The researchers found this type of low-intensity exercise did nothing to reduce the participants' risk of premature death due to heart problems.

Another study at Harvard measured the effects of vigorous and non-vigorous exercise and risk of death. Subjects who performed high-intensity exercise have a lower risk of death than those who performed moderate-intensity exercise.[9]

To live healthier longer, practice a progressive interval exercise program such as PACE.

That's also what a recent study published in the *Annals of Internal Medicine* found. Researchers followed 644 patients with heart failure over a 10-year period. They found that the heart's peak ventilatory oxygen uptake (VO2) (meaning the heart's exercise capacity) was the most important criteria in predicting chronic heart failure. Exercise capacity was more important than the duration of time exercised in extending life.[10]

What can you do to increase your heart's exercise capacity? Simple: Challenge your capacity, a little bit at first, but as you become conditioned, you can gradually increase the challenge. In other words, you need to perform progressive interval exercise, such as the PACE™ program. Long-duration walking or jogging does little to improve your cardiovascular health. To strengthen your heart and live longer, pick up the pace and follow the PACE™ Program.

Build Muscle Mass with Effective Interval Workouts

Your age doesn't have to dictate your level of fitness or your muscle mass. Sure, if you don't challenge your muscles they will shrink. Without effective exercise, you lose about 3 pounds of muscle every decade after age 30, but you can maintain 100 percent of your youthful muscle mass if you do the right exercises.

Why bother? Because healthy muscle is essential. Your muscle mass is intimately connected to your metabolism in many ways:

- Muscle helps you fight fatigue, sexual dysfunction, chronic illness, sagging skin, and bone fractures.
- Muscles help increase your metabolic rate, which leaves you less susceptible to fat gain.
- Muscles provide energy by storing glycogen.
- Conditioned muscles strengthen the immune system, decreasing your risk of developing disease.
- Muscles help maintain glucose balance.
- Muscle allows you to perform the activities of daily living. Loss of muscle is a major cause of nursing home institutionalization among elderly Americans.

Many people fail to appreciate the continuing need for muscle. If you believe that once you've reached your 60s, 70s or beyond muscle is no longer important, think again! An ongoing study known as the Evergreen Project is studying the effects of muscle on the aging process. The study includes men and women between the ages of 65 and 94. The researchers have already found that those participants with greater muscle mass have better mental function, fewer chronic illnesses, and live longer.[11]

Fortunately, you're never too old to enjoy the benefits of the right exercise. The Human Nutritional Research Center on Aging at Tufts University studied the effect of muscle building exercise on people between the ages of 63 and 98. Most of the study participants required walking aids or wheelchairs. Within 10 weeks, all the participants experienced a notable increase in muscle, as well as improvement in stamina and stability. More importantly, many participants were able to walk unaided after the muscle building exercise therapy.[12]

Keep your muscles strong. Use resistance training to increase lean muscle and regular calisthenics for functional strength.

Create Your Special Exercise Plan

Despite the data, cardiologists rarely prescribe the right exercise to their patients.[13] Don't assume that your doctor's neglect minimizes the power of exercise to transform your heart. By the time you finish chapter 7, Build a Strong Heart: Get More With Less, you'll know how to put into practice an effective exercise plan to stave off or reverse heart disease. You will learn how to work out effectively to build and maintain cardiovascular health. And, remember, you can get fit and stay fit in only about 10 or 15 minutes a day.

Footnotes Chapter 2

1 Sesso HD, Paffenbarger RS Jr and Lee IM. Physical activity and coronary heart disease in men: The Harvard Alumni Health Study. *Circulation.* 2000 Aug. 29; 102(9):975-980.

2 Murphy M, Neville A, Neville C, et al. Accumulating brisk walking for fitness, cardiovascular risk, and psychological health. *Medical and Science for Sports and Exercise.* 2002 Sep; 34(9):1468-1474.

3 Kraemer WJ, Hakkinen K, Newton RU, et al. Effects of heavy-resistance training on hormonal response patterns in younger vs. older men. *Journal of Applied Physiology.* 1999 Sep; 87(3):982-992.

4 Sanchez-Quesada J., et al. Increase of LDL susceptibility to oxidation occurring after intense, long duration aerobic exercise. *Atherosclerosis.* 1995 Dec; 111(2): 297-305.

5 Siegel A, Lewandrowski EL, Chun, KY, et al. Changes in cardiac markers including B-natriuretic peptide in runners after the Boston Marathon. *American Journal of Cardiology.* 2001 Oct 15; 88(8):920-923.

6 Osterberg KL and Melby CL. Effect of acute resistance exercise on postexercise oxygen consumption and resting metabolic rate in young women. *International Journal of Sport Nutrition and Exercise Metabolism.* 2000 Mar; 10(1):71-81.

7 Tremblay A, Simoneau JA and Bouchard C. Impact of exercise intensity on body fitness and skeletal muscle metabolisms. *Metabolism.* 1994 July; 43(7):814-818.

8 DeBusk RF, Stenestrand U, Sheehan M and Haskell WL. Training effects of long versus short bouts of exercise in healthy subjects. *American Journal of Cardiology.* 1990 Apr 15; 65(15):1010-1013.

9 Lee IM, Hsieh CC, and Paffenbarger RS Jr. Exercise intensity and longevity in men. The Harvard Alumni Health Study. *Journal of the American Medical Association.* 1995 Apr 19; 273(15):1179-1184.

10 Myers J, et al. Clinical hemodynamic and cardiopulmonary exercise test determinants of survival in patients referred for evaluation of heart failure. *Annals of Internal Medicine.* 1998; 129:286-293.

11 Fozard J. Epidemiologists try many ways to show that physical activity is good for seniors' health and longevity. Review special issue of Journal of Aging and Physical Activity: The Evergreen Project. *Experimental Aging Research.* 1999 Apr-Jun; 25(2):175-182.

12 Klatz R. Hormones of Youth. *American Academy of Anti-Aging.* Chicago 1999, p. 47-48.

13 Speed CA and Shapiro LM. Exercise prescription in cardiac disease. *The Lancet.* 2000 Oct 7; 356(9237):1208-1210.

3

Cholesterol:
The Great Red Herring

L et me fill you in on a secret the mainstream medical community doesn't want you to know about: Cholesterol doesn't cause heart disease. While you have undoubtedly been exposed to a lot of cholesterol-bashing propaganda, the evidence proves that neither the cholesterol in your diet nor the cholesterol in your blood can be held responsible for cardiovascular disease.

More importantly, all the focus on cholesterol has been a dangerous distraction from the real causes of heart disease. In this chapter, I will explain the facts about cholesterol, but first I want to share the story of my personal struggle with medicine's interpretation of blood cholesterol.

First Encounter with
Dangerously Low Serum Cholesterol

In 1979 I was 22, fresh out of undergraduate school with my whole life ahead of me. I remember how excited I was when I received my letter of acceptance into a medical technology internship program – and how disappointed I was when I received another letter two weeks later telling me that I couldn't start after all. The admissions officers had discovered a medical problem in my entrance physical records. The letter asked me to report to Tampa General Hospital for a meeting with the director of the pathology department.

When I entered his office, the chief pathologist was sitting at his desk, shuffling though papers, and talking into a cassette recorder. He didn't look up but motioned for me to sit. He asked me if I took drugs or drank alcohol. I said, "Alcohol, a little, but only at parties." (I was glad he didn't ask how often I went to parties.) He then asked if anyone in my family had a number of diseases with names I had never heard before. He told me that he was ordering a biopsy of my liver and not to worry about the bill. When I asked him why I needed a biopsy of my liver, he said my liver wasn't making enough cholesterol. "What?" I responded in disbelief.

"Cholesterol, it's a fat in your blood," he explained. "Your blood level is supposed to be from 150 to 300, and yours is only 95. There's something wrong with your liver."

"Oh, I know what cholesterol is," I replied. "My cholesterol is low because I've been a vegetarian for years. I've made it drop lower now because I've been in a very intensive athletic training program."

At this point he wheeled his chair from behind his desk, put his cigarette in an ashtray, leaned forward as his huge belly hung over his chair, and looked at me over bifocals for the first time. "Oh, no son," he said, "exercise won't affect your cholesterol level."

With the help of letters from the Dean of The College of Natural Science and the Director of Athletics at The University of South Florida, who knew me and vouched for my acceptable health, I did get into the internship program without a liver biopsy. But for decades to follow, my view would continue to differ from the widely accepted beliefs about what blood cholesterol levels mean.

Serum Cholesterol Is Innocent!

Your cholesterol blood level can tell you useful information about your health and fitness, but it is not the great predictor of heart disease that conventional medicine leads us to believe. In fact, these numbers make very poor crystal balls, as I learned from experience.

Years ago, I began inheriting a group of patients who "dropped out" with other doctors because they refused to lower their cholesterol levels. These cantankerous old men didn't trust doctors and weren't willing to change their lifestyles in ways that seemed to contradict their instincts.

Over the years, I noticed that these rebels with high cholesterol rarely had heart problems. Recently, the University Hospital in Switzerland announced that they did not find a statistically significant link between cholesterol and coronary artery disease. Clearly, cholesterol isn't the ultimate heart attack warning it was made out to be.

When you look past your preconceived notions about health and examine the evidence, the facts are clear: Nearly 75 percent of people who have heart attacks have normal cholesterol levels.[1] Turns out, the maverick patients were right not to take everything their doctors said as gospel. We now know that total blood cholesterol levels are very poor predictors of heart attack or stroke. Still, most doctors continue to turn to conventional cholesterol screening as the best predictor of heart attacks.

The Cholesterol Drug Campaign

When doctors see patients' high blood cholesterol levels, they usually prescribe drugs. Every year, conventional doctors write more than 50 million prescriptions for cholesterol-lowering medications, which are toxic and have harmful side effects. Recently the National Cholesterol Education Program (NCEP) issued new guidelines that call for even more aggressive diagnosis and treatment of high cholesterol. About 13 million people take cholesterol-lowering drugs, and that number will triple in the next few years in response to the stricter guidelines.

This policy will have tragic consequences. Drugs are appropriate for short-term use in emergencies, but they are poor substitutes for rooting out underlying causes of chronic disease. Nowhere is this more apparent than with the use of drugs to beat down cholesterol in healthy people. (You can learn more about the dangers of using the commonly prescribed cardiovascular drugs in Chapter 4, America's Heart Drug Problem.)

Once Again Bad Science
Identifies the Wrong Culprit

For the last 50 years, most researchers exploring the causes of heart disease focused on the idea that cardiovascular disease is linked to fat in the diet. As was discussed in the last chapter, this occurred in part because of incomplete population studies that incorrectly compared the modern Western diet to poor Third World diets rather than to the natural diet of our pre-agrarian ancestors. Simply put, this hypothesis holds that a high-fat diet causes high blood cholesterol. High blood cholesterol, in turn, causes atherosclerosis or buildup of plaque in the arteries. Finally, this blockage of the arteries results in a heart attack. This is what your doctor has been telling you, right?

This theory seemed reasonable, except that the underlying presumption that Americans eat a higher fat diet than the historical norm turned out to be contradicted by both the archeological record and evidence from many different surviving hunter-gatherers. But there's another big problem: Even if we presume that we did eat too much fat, no one has ever proved that this causes high cholesterol or that high blood cholesterol causes heart disease. In fact, since the 1950s, truly objective scientific studies repeatedly demonstrate the fallacy of this approach.

We can trace the beginning of this idea linking the amount of fat in the diet to heart disease to a 1953 University of Minnesota study. In this study, Ancel Keys constructed a graph that compared the death rates from heart disease and high total fat intake among people in six countries.[2] From the data he chose to include on the graph, it looked quite convincing.

But there were problems with the study. Dr. Keys used data from only six countries rather than the available data from 22 countries. Why? Because if he had used all the data, the data would not have always showed high death rates from heart disease linked to high total fat intake amounts. For example, the death rate in Finland was seven times the death rate in Mexico, even though people in both countries consumed about the same amount of fat.[3] The bottom line: It proved easier to discard the data from Mexico than to rethink the assumption that dietary fat causes heart disease.

Look at the comparisons in these charts below.

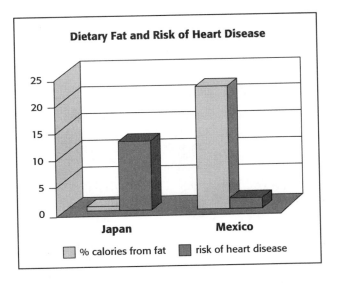

Mexico has 2750 percent higher fat intake than Japan, yet only one-sixth the risk of heart disease. Or, to look at it another way, Japan has the very lowest fat intake of the 22 countries in the study, but a risk of heart disease 600 percent higher than Mexico. Before you decide that this is a peculiar exception unique to Japan, consider the next chart:

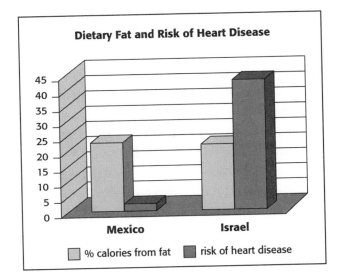

In this chart, Mexico and Israel have nearly identical fat intake, yet Israel has 2100 percent higher risk of heart disease.

Before you think these comparisons are different only because of geography and genetics, look at Finland and Sweden, adjoining North European countries with very similar genetics.

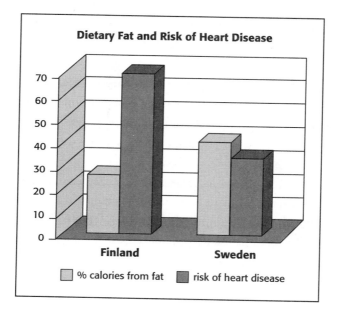

Risk Factors and Causes Are Different

To get a handle on how your dietary fat, your blood cholesterol and your risk of heart disease may be related, it is important to recognize the difference between *risk factors* and *causes*. Risk factors do not necessarily cause disease. This is a crucial difference, one that has often tripped up researchers who study dietary fat and heart disease.

Here is an illustration: When you look at the data, you see that in some of the countries where heart attacks are more common people eat more fat, but they also eat more protein and sugar, they smoke more cigarettes, and they buy more DVD players. Calories from fat tend to be more expensive than calories from other nutrients, so the intake of animal fat becomes statistically associated with deaths from heart disease in affluent countries.

This information simply tells you that heart disease is more common in affluent countries, but it does not prove one thing causes the other.

The truth is that population studies never prove cause and effect. They are useful because population studies can flag important information that we can investigate further. Yet if you chose to ignore the need to prove cause beyond mere association, you could construct a graph that would show that heart attacks, strokes, hypertension, obesity and diabetes are all caused by television sets because there is a direct statistical correlation between the numbers of TV's per household and the rate of these diseases!

When scientists collect and analyze data, they refer to factors that tend to occur at the same time as the disease does as *risk factors*. This conventional naming is somewhat misleading because risk factors don't necessarily convey risks but simply *associations*. As in the above example, owning multiple TV's could be cited as a risk factor for heart attacks, even though owning a TV will not increase your risk of having a heart attack.

There are several hundred risk factors for heart disease, including smoking, high blood pressure, obesity, lack of exercise, stress, male sex, income, race, age, and baldness to name a few. To move beyond risk factors to determine the cause of cardiovascular disease, scientists must carefully design and conduct experiments to prove a direct cause-and-effect relationship. This research has been done, and it does not show a link between the amount of dietary fat and heart disease.

We Ate Less Fat but Heart Attacks Increased

To find out how fat in the diet affects heart attack rate, it is helpful to study how eating patterns have changed to see if the heart attack rate changed, too. If dietary fat caused heart disease, then the heart attack rate would increase when fat intake increases, and it would decrease when fat intake declines. The data simply does not bear this out. (Keep in mind, even if the numbers did link dietary fat and heart disease, it would not necessarily prove that the fat and not some other related factor was the cause of heart disease.)

From World War I to the 1980s, the death rate from heart attack increased while fat intake declined. In the United States, the death rate from cardiovascular disease increased about tenfold between 1930 and 1960.[4] During that time, the consumption of animal fat declined. If the dietary fat model was correct, the heart attack rate should have declined in keeping with the decline in consumption of fat.

Additional studies shoot down this theory. In the 1960s, researchers from Vanderbilt University studied the Masai tribe in Kenya.[5] These slender shepherds drink about a half gallon of whole milk each day, and they feast on as much as four to ten pounds of meat on occasions. If dietary fat caused high cholesterol and heart disease, the Masai would have sky-high lipid levels and high rates of heart disease, but they have neither. The researchers found that the Masai have exceedingly low rates of heart disease and low cholesterol levels, about 50 percent lower than most Americans do.

Other researchers explored changes in cholesterol when the nomadic Masai moved to urban Nairobi and changed their eating habits. They found that the urban dwellers ate *less* animal fat, but their cholesterol levels were 25 percent *higher* than their fat-eating kinsmen were.[6]

Clearly, some people consume large – even huge – amounts of animal fat and maintain extraordinarily low rates of heart disease and low blood cholesterol levels. This evidence alone dispels the belief that heart disease is caused by dietary fat. Still, many doctors refuse to let go of this outdated idea. Most doctors never read the original studies or examine the data that supports this conclusion. When they do, they, too, learn there is no scientific evidence to support the assumption that eating dietary fat causes high cholesterol.

Cholesterol Levels Generally Do Not Predict Heart Attacks

Even if you dismiss the link between dietary fat and cholesterol, you may still be left with the impression that heart disease is caused by high blood cholesterol levels, regardless of whether they are caused by diet or some other factor. Once again, the data does *not* back this claim.

Doctors and drug companies often refer to the famous Framingham study when talking about cardiovascular risk. Framingham is a small town near Boston, where for more than 50 years, researchers have followed the population and tracked risk factors for heart disease. Government organizations often cite these study results as a reason to beat cholesterol into submission, using potent prescription drugs if necessary. But what does the study really reveal?

Amazingly, Framingham researchers themselves reported that "80 percent of heart attack patients had similar lipid levels [i.e., fat levels in the blood] to those who did not have heart attacks."[7] In other words, cholesterol levels do not predict heart attacks in the vast majority of patients. The link between cholesterol and women was essentially nil; women with low cholesterol died just as often as women with high cholesterol. Furthermore, according to data from the Framingham study, almost half of the people in the study who had a heart attack had low cholesterol.

Ironically, as the study participants grew older, the association between cholesterol and heart disease became weaker, not stronger. In fact, according to the data, for men above age 47, cholesterol levels made no difference in cardiovascular mortality.[8] Since 95 percent of all heart attacks occur in people above age 48 – and those who have heart attacks at an earlier age are usually diabetics or have a rare genetic problem – then most people do not have to worry about their cholesterol levels! Remember that even if we could show an association between cholesterol blood levels and heart disease, it would not prove that cholesterol caused heart disease.

Sometimes When Serum Cholesterol Goes Down, Risk of Dying Goes Up

Now another fact to make you wonder what the experts were thinking: High cholesterol seems to have a protective effect in the elderly. According to research done at the Department of Cardiovascular Medicine at Yale University, nearly twice as many people with low cholesterol had heart attacks when compared to those with high cholesterol levels.[9] Data from the Framingham study also supports the finding that when blood cholesterol decreases, the risk of dying actually increases.

There is no question that blood cholesterol is involved in the accumulation of plaque in the arteries. Plaque buildup narrows the arteries and restricts blood flow, often leading to heart attacks and strokes. Yet the conventional approach continues to miss the most important point: the plaque buildup is dangerous, not the presence of cholesterol itself.

What is Cholesterol?
ESSENTIAL INGREDIENT FOR LIFE, HEALTH AND SEX

Although cholesterol has a bad reputation for clogging the arteries, it's not the enemy. Cholesterol is essential for life and health. It provides energy to cells, helps make cell membranes, and assists in the formation of sheaths around nerves. Plus, it plays a vital role in the production of the sex hormones testosterone, estrogen and progesterone, and other adrenal hormones like DHEA and cortisol.

While cholesterol is in some foods we eat, the liver manufactures most of it. In fact, each day our bodies churn out about 1,000 milligrams of cholesterol, compared to the average dietary intake of about 325 milligrams for men or 220 milligrams for women.

No matter whether it comes from the liver or our diet, cholesterol and other dietary fats must move from the digestive system and into the cells to perform these terrific tasks. Fat must be packaged into protein-covered particles that allow the fat to mix with the blood. These tiny particles are lipoproteins (lipid – or fat – plus protein).

Remove Plaque from Arteries Now
By Raising HDL

You've probably heard about the two types of lipoproteins: low-density lipoproteins (LDLs) and high-density lipoproteins (HDLs). LDLs help lay down the plaque deposits in the arteries (that's why this is the "bad" cholesterol), and HDLs help remove plaque from the arteries (that's why this is the "good" cholesterol). The bloodstream carries many sizes and types of lipoproteins. Those with a little fat and lots of protein are heavier and denser; those with more fat are lighter and less dense.

The different types of lipoproteins determine where in the body the bloodstream delivers the fats. While most doctors prescribe traditional cholesterol tests that tell you your total cholesterol, LDL, and HDL levels, these don't reveal enough information to tell whether you are measuring a normal building block for sex hormones or an abnormal heart threat. When it comes to determining healthy cholesterol profiles, doctors need more specific details. You can find out just how to use the details about your blood cholesterol profile in Chapter 5, Measure Your Real Heart Health.

Drug Corporations Profit from Misinformation

Pharmaceutical companies continue to make billions of dollars annually as long as they support the myth that cholesterol causes heart disease. As the previous evidence shows, elevated cholesterol levels do not cause heart attacks, so it is unnecessary to take drugs to lower cholesterol.

Results from numerous independent drug trials also do not support the connection between cholesterol and heart disease. The National Heart, Lung and Blood Institute conducted the Lipid Research Clinics Coronary Primary Prevention Trial to test the effectiveness of cholestyramine, a drug known to lower cholesterol. Seven years later, researchers analyzed the data and found that the cholesterol levels decreased by 8 percent, but there were no important (statistically significant) differences in heart attack rates.[10]

Researchers have summarized all drug trials published before 1994 (the year drug companies introduced statin drugs). These studies found that the number of deaths from heart attack was equal in the treatment and control groups, and the total number of deaths was actually greater in the treatment groups. None of the trials showed any statistically significant decrease in the death rate from coronary disease.[11] What it all boils down to is that these cholesterol-lowering drugs lowered cholesterol, but they did not decrease deaths from heart attack.

Make Room for the Most Profitable Drugs in History

In 1994, drug companies introduced a new class of cholesterol-lowering drugs known as statins. These drugs interfere with the body's production of cholesterol, and they block the production of other essential nutrients, including CoQ10. Studies found that these drugs not only lower blood cholesterol levels but also produced a slightly lowered risk of heart attack.

Before we reach the conclusion that lowering cholesterol caused the modestly lowered heart attack rate, we must note that there was no relationship between the amount of the cholesterol reduction and the amount of the risk reduction. We call this phenomenon "lack of exposure response." What this usually means is that the factor being investigated – in this case cholesterol – is not the true cause, but is secondary to or merely associated with the true cause. Stated another way, statins may reduce heart attack risk, but they do so in some way other than reducing cholesterol.

The drug companies that sponsor these studies are very slick at directing attention away from this failure. Only very recently has it come to light that statins do other things more directly related to heart disease risk, such as lowering the inflammatory blood marker, C-reactive protein. (You can learn more about the role of C-reactive protein in predicting heart disease in Chapter 5.) The "lack of exposure response" may be because statins help by reducing inflammation, not cholesterol.

But there is more to the story. Statins are expensive; a typical dose costs about $1,000 to $1,500 per year. And, more significantly, statins block an antioxidant system important to your cardiovascular health and rob your organs of this crucial nutrient. Statins can make you chronically fatigued and cause muscles aches. They also stimulate cancer growth in rodents. In human studies, breast cancer was more common in women who took the drug than those in the control group.

Additionally, it's wise to cautiously review information from drug studies that pharmaceutical companies fund. These corporations benefit remarkably when research results recommend a new drug. Statins are the most profitable drugs in history. Those profits buy a lot of propaganda, such as lobbyists in Washington, direct-to-consumer advertising, and marketing to doctors, including free continuing medical education about how to prescribe the drugs! This is the fox overseeing the hen house, and the consequences involve your health.

Effective Diet and Exercise, Not Drugs, Restore Heart Health

Once again, many doctors do not study the primary sources. They often do not realize that they are victims of a marketing blitz by the drug companies. Many doctors hear about these studies through carefully crafted press releases from the drug companies or from the drug reps and their brochures. It's easier and faster for a busy doctor to reach for a prescription pad than to take the time to counsel their patients about exercise and diet. It's all too easy for doctors to turn to drug therapy, even though this approach is costly, dangerous, and ineffective in the end. (Discover more compelling reasons to avoid these drugs in the next chapter.)

Lower Your Heart Disease Risk by Raising Good Cholesterol

What traditional cholesterol measure, if any, is important to monitor for heart health? The answer is HDL, the so-called "good" cholesterol. HDL is the single most important cholesterol factor in determining your risk of developing heart disease. Don't worry about lowering your total cholesterol level or your LDL level, just raise your HDL cholesterol.

The Framingham study shows that high levels of HDL are directly related to lower risk of heart disease. In fact, it showed that increased HDL could reduce coronary disease independent of LDL cholesterol.[12] This is the real eye-opener: If your HDL is above 85, you are at no greater risk of heart disease if your total cholesterol is 350 than if it's 150.

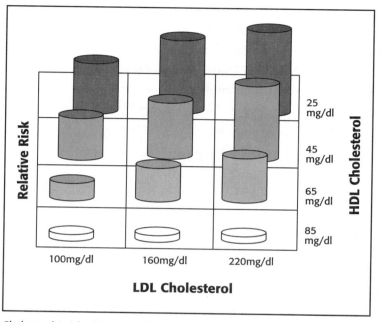

Cholesterol & risk of Coronary Heart Disease
From Framingham Heart Study

High HDLs trump other cholesterol concerns. Why isn't this simple and powerful advice getting through? For one reason, there is no drug to boost HDL. What's the best way to increase HDL cholesterol? Exercise. (You can learn how to raise your HDL cholesterol with exercise in Chapter 7, Build a Strong Heart: Get More with Less.)

Low Serum Cholesterol Levels Are Dangerous to Your Health

Drug companies got a recent boost in sales when the National Cholesterol Education Program published new cholesterol guidelines, which dictate that almost everyone needs cholesterol-lowering drugs. According to the guidelines, the optimal cholesterol levels are below 130 for LDL and below 200 for total cholesterol.

The new recommendations advise that you take steps to even further lower your cholesterol levels if you have any risk factors for cardiovascular disease. Risk factors include a history of cardiovascular disease, high blood pressure, and smoking. This you-can-never-be-too-rich-or-have-too-low-a-cholesterol-level approach backfires when you look at the consequences of very low cholesterol levels. Studies have linked pushing cholesterol levels below 160 to depression and low testosterone levels.

In 2000, Dutch researchers found that men with low cholesterol levels had an increased risk of depression[13]. Cholesterol may affect the metabolism of the mood-altering substance known as serotonin. Other studies have found that serotonin levels are lower in men with low levels of cholesterol. It appears that cholesterol levels below 160 may be low enough to put men at risk.

Restore Heart Health by Using Ways That Work

I told you my cholesterol level in 1979 was an exceptionally low 95. The obese pathologist was wrong when he claimed that exercise couldn't affect cholesterol levels; he was wrong when he claimed that I had liver disease, but he was right about one thing. It is unhealthy to have a cholesterol level that low. This taught me very early in my experience with cholesterol that low serum cholesterol levels are dangerous to your health. It is particularly unhealthy to artificially drive cholesterol down with drugs.

Without knowing the real dangers, I lowered my cholesterol levels without drug therapy by avoiding all animal products for years while following an aggressive multi-sport training regimen. But I did not escape the harmful consequences of excessively low cholesterol. I began losing body hair and libido, and I found my strength failing in gymnastics. I diagnosed myself as having low testosterone (remember, our bodies make testosterone from cholesterol). To correct the problem, I began eating fish and eggs. It would be years later before I knew enough to begin eating red meat again. I also decreased the duration of my training programs. The recovery in my strength and sex drive was almost immediate.

Today, my cholesterol level ranges from 170 to 200, and my HDL cholesterol level is consistently above 100. These do not have to be your measures, and in Chapter 5 you'll identify optimal ranges for various indicators for heart health. I am confident that I have a very low risk for heart disease. I feel stronger, more energetic, more virile, and healthier than I did when my cholesterol was very low.

I am happy to report that I was able to overcome the harmful effects of bad advice, and you can, too. In fact, the sooner you begin the more life, vitality and heart health you'll enjoy!

Footnotes Chapter 3

1 Castelli WP. Cholesterol and lipids in the risk of coronary artery disease-- the Framingham Heart Study. *Canadian Journal of Cardiology*. 1998 July; 4 Suppl A:5A-10A.

2 Keys A. Atherosclerosis: A problem in newer public health. *Journal of Mount Sinai Hospital*. 1953; 20,118-139.

3 Ravnskov U. *The Cholesterol Myths*. New Trends Publishing, Inc.: Wash-ington, D.C.. 2000; pp. 16-19.

4 Keys A. Atherosclerosis: A problem in newer public health. *Journal of Mount Sinai Hospital*. 1953; 20,118-139.

5 Mann G.V., et al. Cardiovascular disease in the Masai. *Journal of Atherosclerosis Research*. 1964; 4:289-312.

6 Day J, et al. Anthropometric, physiological and biochemical differences between urban and rural Maasai. *Atherosclerosis*. 1976; 23:357-361.

7 Gordon T, Castelli WP, Hjortland MC, et al. High density lipoprotein as a positive factor against coronary heart disease. The Framingham Study. *American Journal of Medicine*. 1997 May; 62(5):707-714.

8 Ravnskov U. *The Cholesterol Myths*. New Trends Publishing, Inc.: Wash-ington, D.C.. 2000; p. 56.

9 Krumholz HM, Seeman TE, Merrill SS, et al. Lack of association between cholesterol and coronary heart disease mortality and morbidity and all-cause mortality in persons older than 70 years. *Journal of the American Medical Association*. 1994 Nov; 272(17):1335-1340.

10 [No authors listed] The Lipid Research Clinics Coronary Primary Prevention Trial results. I. Reduction in incidence of coronary heart disease. *Journal of the American Medical Association.* 1984 Jan 20; 251(3):351-64.

11 Ravnskov U. Cholesterol-lowering trials in coronary heart disease: frequency of citation and outcome. *British Journal of Medicine.* 1992 July 4; 305(6844): 15-19.

12 Castiglioni A and Neuman, WR. HDL Cholesterol: What is its true clinical significance?. *Emergency Medicine.*, 2003 Jan; 4(1):30-42.

13 Speed CA and Shapiro LM. Exercise prescription in cardiac disease. *The Lancet.* 2000 Oct 7; 356(9237):1208-1210.

4

America's Heart Drug Problem

Y̲ou should expect to feel better after receiving treatment from a doctor, but many prescription medications recommended for heart disease can make your symptoms worse. Almost all cardiologists prescribe drugs to their heart attack patients. They do this because studies show that drugs reduce the risk of repeat heart attacks, but are they the only way – or even the best way – to lower heart attack risk? No. In truth, drugs often make patients feel worse and their side effects can interfere with more important rehabilitation efforts.

A friend from college recently had a heart attack. When Roy G. came to me for help, he said, "If this is what it's like to survive a heart attack, I'd rather die." He was among the lucky 50 percent who survive their first heart attacks, but his suffering was prolonged and severe. Roy had no prior knowledge that he had heart disease and was not yet 50 years old. The experience scared Roy, and he strictly followed every bit of his doctor's advice. Unfortunately, the doctor's only recommendations were to take medications. Each of the drugs created additional health problems for Roy, interfering with his rehabilitation and the reconditioning of his damaged heart.

Roy's cardiologist first gave him a Nitro patch. It made him feel tired, with chronic low-grade headaches. His prescriptions also included two blood pressure drugs, Altace and Lopressor; despite the drugs, Roy's blood pressure remained high at 180/100. These drugs made him tired and gave him intermittent impotence.

Roy's cholesterol level was 219. His doctor prescribed Lipitor, a statin drug used to lower cholesterol. Roy's total cholesterol declined when he went on the drug, but his HDL (good) cholesterol dropped as well, actually increasing his cholesterol risk ratio.

Roy's reaction? "That drug gave me such terrible pain in my back and legs that I could hardly get out of bed." He said, "It made me feel like I was 80 years old."

I worked to wean Roy from the prescription drugs. The first to go was Lipitor. Roy reported, "The constant pain in my muscles vanished within days of stopping the drug." Roy balanced his cholesterol with diet, exercise, and the natural supplement Policosanol.

Next, Roy quit taking the beta-blocker Lopressor, and his constant fatigue disappeared. "All that time I thought I was so damn tired all the time because I had had a heart attack," Roy said. "It turns out it was the drugs they started me on in the hospital. I was always so weak that I just couldn't exercise." Exercise is a vital component to rehabilitating an injured heart.

With his energy coming back, Roy agreed to commit to both interval and strength training. At the time of his heart attack, Roy weighed 235 pounds and had 30 percent body fat. Within months, he dropped to 205 pounds with a much healthier 20 percent body fat. At last report, Roy was at his goal weight of 185 pounds with 16 percent body fat.

More importantly, Roy's heart became stronger. His original stress test after the heart attack showed significant damage to the heart. A second stress test done three months later showed marked improvement, with damage rated as mild. A third stress test showed minimal damage, and the reporting cardiologist said it was difficult to see any evidence that Roy had ever had a heart attack.

Roy's Progress

	Heart Attack	Now
Weight	235	185
% Body Fat	30%	17%
Blood Pressure	160/100	100/65
Resting Heart Rate	100	60
Cholesterol	216	165
LDL Cholesterol	140	90
HDL Cholesterol	40	55
Cardiac Risk Ratio	5.4	2.9
Ventricular Ejection Fraction	49%	60%

Note the last row in the table above. Your ejection fraction is the percentage of blood received that your heart pumps back out with each beat. It is a measure of youth and strength in your heart. Most experts consider it impossible to strengthen the heart after a cardiac episode, but Roy proved them wrong.

Roy's experience with drugs to treat heart disease is quite common. In this chapter, you'll see how each of the categories of drugs taken by millions of people with cardiovascular problems – including cholesterol-lowering drugs, blood-pressure-lowering drugs, and other cardiac medications – often do more harm than good.

While you, like Roy, may be better off without taking your prescription medications, *never stop taking your prescription medications without the guidance of your physician.* There can be harmful results when you suddenly quit taking some medications. Be sure you have effective professional support when you decide to go this route. Fortunately, there are steps you can take to strengthen your heart, without turning to prescription medications. In Chapter 11, Individualize Your *Doctor's Heart Cure,* you will discover drug-free steps to lower your cholesterol and blood pressure.

Go Natural
IT'S SAFER, EASIER ON YOUR BODY, AND MORE ECONOMICAL

For chronic health problems, there are natural alternatives to prescription drugs. These substances are safer and have fewer dangerous side effects than prescription drugs, which can burden your kidneys and liver when you take them for a long time. In addition, natural remedies are more economical. Prescription drugs are expensive. Drug manufacturers pocket the profit and pass the costs along to you.

Of course, prescription drugs play an essential role in your health care. The appropriate medication can save your life when you face an emergency or an acute medical problem. Fortunately, most prescription drugs for long-term problems have effective, inexpensive natural alternatives. If you are taking prescription drugs, ask your doctor about the alternatives. If he won't tell you about alternatives, it may be time to consult a new doctor.

Stay Away From Statin Cholesterol-Lowering Drugs if You Can

Most doctors readily prescribe cholesterol-lowering drugs called statins. The US Food and Drug Administration reports that 20 million Americans currently take these drugs. They are the most commonly prescribed drugs for lowering cholesterol. The National Cholesterol Education Program estimates that this number could triple in response to the government's new guidelines for cholesterol management.

Statin drugs do lower cholesterol levels, but not without devastating side effects, such as liver toxicity, digestive tract upset, rashes, blurred vision, muscle inflammation and weakness, and a rarely discussed but potentially lethal side effect known as *rhabdomyolysis*. This horrific complication occurs when the drug causes the smooth muscle cells to burst and dump their contents into the bloodstream. This can then overwhelm the kidneys as they work to clear the cellular debris, resulting in kidney failure and death.

The Food and Drug Administration reports at least 81 deaths from this complication of statin drugs since 1997. In 2001, Bayer withdrew Baycol – one of the more popular statin drugs – from the market after at least 31 people died due to complication from rhabdomyolysis. Fifty additional deaths from this single side effect occurred in people using the other five statin drugs still on the market – Lescol, Lipitor, Mevacor, Pravachol, and Zocor. These five drugs are also associated with the more common side effect of liver toxicity, especially in the elderly.

In addition to putting you at risk for rhabdomyolysis and liver problems, statin drugs have another side effect that happens in every person who takes them. Through their primary action, statin drugs block the body's production of CoQ10, a nutrient essential for heart health. CoQ10 is an important energizing nutrient and antioxidant protector for the heart. Studies have found that statins deplete the body of CoQ10 by as much as 40 percent. By the time you read Chapter 8, Energize the Heart: The Miracle of CoQ10, you'll realize why this is so detrimental to heart health.

Politics, Pills, and Profits

What makes doctors prescribe medications – with such terrifying side effects – so often? Lipitor and Zocor have been among the 10 most profitable prescription drugs since 1999, raking in $9.2 billion in sales. Slick advertising campaigns and promotions fool physicians by sensationalizing the benefits and downplaying the harmful side effects. These drugs appear to offer a quick fix for people with high cholesterol.

Statin drugs do lower cholesterol levels, sometimes without a patient making any changes in diet or exercise. Many doctors find it easier to reach for the prescription pad than to take the time to explain the importance of diet and appropriate supplements. They also fail to research or remain open-minded about the safe, effective, and inexpensive alternatives to statin drugs that can lower cholesterol and reduce heart risks without dangerous side effects.

If you are currently taking statin drugs, ask your doctor for an alternative. If you must take one of these drugs, insist that you have your liver function monitored with a blood test every three months. If there is any sign of liver toxicity, stop taking the drug.

If you develop muscle pain, fatigue, or tenderness (particularly in the calves or back), notify your doctor immediately. Also, let your doctor know if you develop a fever or dark urine. You may need a blood test to detect the presence of a muscle enzyme known as creatine kinase, which is elevated when a person develops rhabdomolysis.

Is Drug Research Biased?
SLICK MARKETING DISGUISED AS SCIENCE, SELLS DRUGS

Do you know drug companies pay for the studies that show benefits from their drugs? Drug manufacturers sponsor research that makes them look good.

Consider the case of the Pfizer-sponsored research on Lipitor, a drug to lower cholesterol levels. Pfizer funded a trial in which 20,000 participants (not all of whom had elevated cholesterol levels) took either Lipitor or a placebo. The researchers found that people in the Lipitor group experienced a lowering of their cardiac risk, even if their cholesterols were normal. Pfizer stopped the study before researchers completed it because, Pfizer argued, it would be unfair to deny Lipitor to the placebo group.[1] Scientists implied that Lipitor offers such significant health benefits that they recommended it even for patients with normal cholesterol levels.

Remember the side effects? The study never mentions them. The *Physicians' Desk Reference* lists the side effects of Lipitor, including liver dysfunction and failure, kidney failure, rhabdomyolysis, constipation, insomnia, tinnitus, and high blood pressure. Yes, the drug designed to protect the heart by lowering cholesterol levels can threaten the heart by causing high blood pressure! Despite the apparent conflict, the study recommends that doctors prescribe

Lipitor to patients with hypertension even if their cholesterol levels are already normal. The bulk of the evidence does not support this approach.

The study also fails to mention additional dangers associated with statin drugs. For example, a Finnish study found that statin drugs decrease antioxidant levels by as much as 22 percent (that means harmful oxidation increases). Another study showed Zocor increases insulin levels by 13 percent, increasing the risk of heart disease, hypertension, obesity, insulin resistance, and Type 2 diabetes.[2]

There is a troubling complacency in the medical profession that allows drug-company-sponsored research to dominate respected medical journals. When looking at research, don't take the conclusions at face value. The drug and research corporations do not always reveal serious, even deadly, problems with prescription medications. Read the results with a skeptical eye. Don't be afraid to question whether there is a safer way of achieving the same desired results – without dependence on dangerous prescription drugs.

Don't Pay Dearly for Blood Pressure Drugs

The big drug companies may have duped your doctor about the effectiveness of their most popular blood pressure medication, and you may be paying the price with a needlessly increased risk of heart attack and death. In addition, as described below, you also may pay up to 900 percent more for a new generation of drugs that are less effective than the older ones.

About 20 years ago, doctors began using two new classes of drugs to treat high blood pressure: calcium channel blockers and ACE inhibitors.

- Calcium channel blockers: Calcium channel blockers (also known as calcium antagonists) enter the channels in the smooth muscle cells of the arteries, causing the arteries to relax and dilate. This reduces blood pressure and improves circulation, often while slowing the heart rate. These drugs include nifedipine (Adalat CC, Procardia XL), verapamil

(Calan SR, Covera HS, Isoptin SR, and Verelan), and diltiazem (Cardizem CD, Cardizem SR, Dilacor XR, and Tiazac), and there are more. Side effects include headache, flushing, constipation, nausea, elevated cholesterol, edema (fluid retention), and low blood pressure. More importantly, studies find that people taking calcium channel blockers actually experienced a 60 percent increase in heart attack compared to people who used other blood pressure medications.[3]

- ACE Inhibitors: Angiotensin-converting enzyme (ACE) inhibitors are often used to treat high blood pressure and congestive heart failure (condition where the heart cannot keep up with the blood and the body retains too much fluid, often causing legs and ankles to swell, and congestion in the lungs). These drugs work by causing the arteries to relax and dilate slightly. Blood pressure falls, oxygen demands decrease, and the heart pumps more blood. These drugs include ramipril (Altace), quinapril (Accupril), captopril (Capoten), lisinopril (Prinivil and Zestril), and benazepril (Lotensin), among others. The most common side effect of ACE inhibitors is a dry cough. Additional side effects include reduced appetite, mineral deficiencies, kidney damage, and reduced white blood cell count.

Safer, Cheaper, Better but Ignored

Drug companies said these were better than the traditional treatment of water pills (diuretics), and doctors believed them. Over the last decade, prescriptions of these new drugs have soared. But now a very large study sponsored by the National Heart, Lung, and Blood Institute proved the two classes of drugs are actually far less effective than diuretics. In a disturbing twist, all the original evidence supporting the effectiveness of the drugs seems to have disappeared.

The stakes here are huge. One out of four Americans suffers from high blood pressure. By getting doctors to switch from affordable water pills to expensive new drugs to treat the problem, drug companies generate billions of dollars in new business. The following chart compares the monthly cost of the various treatments for high blood pressure:

Monthly Cost Comparisons

Brand Name	Generic	Manufacturer	Cost/Mo.
CALCIUM CHANNEL BLOCKERS			
Cardizem SR	Diltiazem	Biovail	$96.98
Norvasc	Amiodipine	Pfizer	$68.09
Procardia XL	Nifedipine	Pfizer	$93.59
Verelan	Verapamil	Schwarz Pharma	$122.99
ACE INHIBITORS			
Prinvil	Lisinopril	Merck	$62.99
Zestril	Lisinopril	AstraZeneca	$61.29
Vasotec	Enalapri Maleate	Biovail	$56.94
DIURETICS			
HCTZ	Hydorchlorothiazide	Generics	$7.99
Dyazide	Triamterne	GlaxoSmithKline	$14.89
Lasix	Furosemide	Aventis	$9.99

As the table shows, diuretics cost only pennies a day and are, on average, about one-tenth as expensive as the newer calcium channel blockers like Cardizem. And, as the recent research has proven, these very inexpensive drugs are more effective than the high-priced competitors at lowering blood pressure. What convinced thousands of doctors to recommend the new drugs? The drug corporations' million-dollar marketing campaigns – instead of solid, valid, reliable research – sold physicians on the new drugs. As mentioned earlier, drug manufacturers aggressively advertise directly to doctors. Appealing sales reps visit doctors and bring free samples, pens, prescription pads, calculators, and clocks. They also bring lavish gifts such as $100 gift certificates, free stethoscopes, paid conferences, dinners, and tickets to major sporting events. The strategy has paid off. Sales of the new drugs grossed over $10 billion for the drug companies.

Doctors with Financial Ties
Write More Prescriptions

After doctors switched millions of patients to high-priced new drugs without evidence of superior effectiveness, a massive, well-controlled study proved that these new, expensive drugs are not as effective as simple, old-fashioned water pills. In a double-blind, collaborative study by 623 heart health centers, 42,000 subjects took either a diuretic, calcium channel blocker, or an ACE inhibitor. Researchers then monitored these patients over a five-year period. The results, reported in the December 2002 issue of the *Journal of the American Medical Association*, unequivocally concluded that diuretics are the best treatment. Patients taking Zestril or Prinivil, for instance, had a 19 percent higher risk of heart disease than those taking diuretics. Those taking Norvasc had a 38 percent higher risk of heart failure.

In addition to identifying the best treatment, the study also reveals the problems with how doctors choose treatment options. Doctors switched to the new drugs even though diuretics have long had a more proven track record and cost up to 90 percent less. A study published in *The New England Journal of Medicine* showed that *96 percent of articles in medical journals that supported the use of calcium channel blockers were written by doctors with financial ties to the drug maker.* This landmark study underscores the reason drug company information is untrustworthy, and why you should strive to minimize the use of drugs whenever possible.

Warnings for Water Pills, Too

Diuretics may be better and cheaper than other blood pressure medications, but they come with their own list of unwanted side effects. The most common group of water pills known as thiazide diuretics raise total cholesterol, LDL (bad) cholesterol, and triglyceride levels. Other side effects include:

- Weakness
- Sensitivity to light
- Dehydration
- Gouty arthritis
- Decreased sexual desire

- Muscle cramps
- Diarrhea
- Joint pain
- Vomiting

Fortunately, you can lower your blood pressure naturally, without relying on diuretics or other prescription medication. More than half of the patients treated at the Center for Health and Wellness who used to take blood pressure drugs have been able to stop taking those drugs while keeping their blood pressure down with the nutrient, CoQ10. In Chapter 11, you'll learn how to lower your blood pressure without using diuretics or prescription medications.

Say "No" to Nitrate-Based Cardiac Drugs if You Can

If you have high blood pressure or chest pain, your doctor probably prescribed a nitrate-based heart medication. Millions of Americans take these drugs, which doctors have prescribed for more than a century. These medications go by names such as Nitroglycerin, Isosorbide, Nitro-Bid, Nitrostat, Nitro-Dur, Imdur, Nitrolingula, Isosorbide, Isoptin, Isordil, Ismo, Dilatrate, and Minitran. Doctors typically prescribe Nitroclycerin, Isosorbide, and Nitro-Bid for chest pain, and other such as Isoptin, Isordil, and Minitran for high blood pressure. The medications may be taken as tiny tablets that you place under your tongue or pills to swallow or patches to wear on the skin.

Do nitrates help to ease chest pain and lower blood pressure? Yes, they do. They temporarily open blood vessels and allow blood to flow back into the heart. With nitrate-based medications, an enzyme in the body breaks down the nitrates into nitric-oxide molecules, which then force open the blood vessels in the body.

The problem with nitrates is that they damage the sensitive lining of the heart and blood vessels known as the endothelium. The endothelium consists of a single layer of thin, flat cells that line internal body cavities.

People with endothelial dysfunction often suffer from heart attacks. In fact, a new study shows these drugs actually more than triple your risk of having a heart attack.

A recent Japanese study shows how damaging nitrates can be. Researchers studied more than 500 participants for almost 4 years and found that subjects who took nitrates on a regular basis were 2.4 times more likely to have a major cardiac event than those who didn't take the drugs.[4] Investigators discovered that the nitrate drugs not only damaged the heart lining, they accelerated any damage already present in the heart.

Fortunately, patients can take natural substances to get nitric oxide into the blood, without causing harmful side effects. To determine whether these safe supplements are for you, refer to Chapter 11 carefully.

Beware the Beta Blockers

Doctors prescribe beta blockers for chest pain, high blood pressure, and congestive heart failure. These drugs attach to the beta adrenergic receptors in the heart and blood vessels, blocking their response to norepinephrine, a hormone that tells the arteries to tighten and the heart to speed up. These drugs lower blood pressure by slowing the heart and relaxing the blood vessels.

Beta blockers can provide temporary relief, but doctors often prescribe them for long-term treatment. These drugs have serious side effects, including fatigue, dizziness, insomnia, nausea, depression, loss of libido, impotence, and cold extremities. Equally concerning, beta blockers can raise triglyceride levels and lower HDL cholesterol. When this happens, these patients are usually then given another drug to counteract this drug-induced side effect. In people with congestive heart failure, beta blockers can actually make the problem worse.

While it may be a good idea to stop taking beta blockers, it is vitally important to wean yourself from them carefully and gradually *under your doctor's supervision.* You can cause serious problems when you suddenly stop taking beta blockers. The "rebound effect" occurs because your body responds to blocking these receptors by building more of them. Going cold turkey causes you to have a greater beta effect than you did before you started the drug. This can cause high blood pressure, chest pain, palpitations, and anxiety, even if you didn't have any of these symptoms before you started the drug.

Drug Giant Knocks Safe Supplement Off the US Market

If you believe the advertising hype, drug companies are benevolent organizations that labor tirelessly to produce pharmaceuticals to improve the health and well-being of all mankind. Don't be naïve. Drug companies do almost anything to manipulate the marketplace in favor of their products.

Consider the marketing of red yeast rice, a product made by fermenting yeast on rice. People in China used this remedy for hundreds of years, and in April 1998, the University of California at Los Angeles School of Medicine published a study showing that red yeast significantly lowers cholesterol levels.

In the United States, a small company called Pharmanex sold red yeast rice as a cholesterol-lowering nutritional supplement known as Cholestin. They had accumulated 13 studies showing red yeast rice lowers cholesterol while being virtually free of serious side effects. Merck, the manufacturer of the cholesterol-lowering prescription drug Mevacor, didn't appreciate the competition. Merck sued Pharmanex, claiming that the natural red yeast rice contains the same compound as Mevacor, thus violating their patent.

According to extensive chemical analysis, the active ingredients are similar, but not identical. Furthermore, Cholestin's active ingredient (mevinolin) occurs naturally, while Mevacor's active ingredient (lovastatin) is produced in a laboratory.[5] Since the law created patents to protect new inventions rather than works of nature, the judge in the case recognized that the products' similarity challenges Mevacor's patent. The active ingredient in red yeast rice occurred naturally before Mevacor was developed. Therefore, the judge ruled that Merck could not interfere with the sale of Cholestin.

Win one for the good guys. But Merck, funded with billions of dollars from the sales of Mevacor and other drugs, appealed – and lost. So they appealed again – and lost. After the third appeal and third denial, another judge warned Merck to stop harassing the smaller company and trying to put it out of business with ongoing legal fees.

Unfortunately, Merck managed to get a different district court to hear the case for a fourth time. In March 2001, the US District Court ruled that Cholestin contained the same active ingredient as Mevacor, concluding that distributors could no longer sell Cholestin in the United States. The Food and Drug Administration enforced the ban, and sent threatening letters to supplement manufacturers. As a result of this unfair drug scandal, red yeast rice is banned from the US market, although you can still find it in some health food stores and on the Internet.

Take Special Care As You Age

As you age, your ability to tolerate medication changes. A medication that you may have been taking for years without problems may eventually poison you as your body becomes less adept at handling it.

With any medication, your liver must detoxify the drug and your kidneys must eliminate it. Drug dosing is based in part on the body's ability to safely remove this toxic burden. When you grow older, your liver and kidneys slow down and become less efficient at processing drugs. If you are removing less of the drug and still taking the same amount, the medicines gradually build up in your body, potentially leading to drug overdose.

Symptoms of overmedication often show up as fatigue, confusion, dizziness, weakness, memory loss, loss of balance, impotence, and constipation – all symptoms that many doctors simply attribute to growing older. The problem is quite widespread. Researchers at Harvard Medical School reviewed the medical records of 6,171 people over 65 and found that 23.5 percent of the participants were being given drugs at doses deemed unsafe for elders.[6]

It's vitally important to protect yourself from overdosing. Once again, it is essential to have good communication with your doctor. Here are some important questions to ask about your medication:

- What is this drug supposed to do?
- What are the alternatives to this medication?
- Is this dose suitable for someone my age? My weight and size?
- How long is it safe to take this medication?
- What are the possible side effects of the medication?
- What are the symptoms of overmedication?
- Does this drug interact with other medications?
- Are there any special precautions with the medication?

Be sure to write down any relevant information about the drug, especially if you are taking more than one medication at a time. Let your doctor know if you lose or gain weight, since bodyweight can have an impact on dosage requirements.

If you think you may be overmedicated, talk to your doctor about your concerns. In many cases, your doctor can perform tests to determine if your liver or kidneys are being overworked or whether the medication is causing other unwanted side effects. Don't be shy about asking for dosage testing; it's a prudent method that may allow you to find out if your body is handling the drug well before dangerous side effects accumulate.

Footnotes Chapter 4

1 Reuters News, Oct 10, 2002.

2 Thompson J. Bias in Reporting on Statins. Health Sciences Institute e-Alert, Oct 31, 2002. http://hsibaltimore.com/ea2002/ea_02131.shtml

3 Psaty B, Heckbert SR, Koepsell TD, et al. The risk of myocardial infarction associated with antihypertensive drug therapies. *Journal of the American Medical Association.* 1995 Aug 23; 274(8):620-625.

4 Circulation Supplement II, Circulation 2002 Nov; 106(19): Preliminary Abstract 1494. (Weil, A., "The Cholestin Controversy," Self Healing 1999, Aug. p. 8)

5 Weil Andrew, "The Cholestin Controversy," Self Healing 1999, Aug. p. 8.

6 Willcox SM, Himmelstein DU and Woolhandler S. Inappropriate drug prescribing for the community dwelling elderly. *Journal of the American Medical Association.* 1994 Jul 27; 272(4): 292-296.

5

Measure Your Real
Heart Health

Y ou probably know very little about the condition of your heart. Your doctor may have performed tests designed to detect certain heart diseases, but these standard tests provide very little information about the capacity, vitality, and strength of your heart.

Fortunately, there are tests that can help you assess your cardiovascular health. By the time you complete this chapter, you'll know how you can use blood tests and other markers to assess your cardiovascular health. These tests do more than tell you whether your heart is normal or diseased; they help you quantify your overall heart health. They let you know where you are doing well and what you need to improve. You can then use these same tests as a scale to track your progress in your heart improvement program.

These tests are easy and inexpensive, yet most doctors don't routinely use them. Don't be shy about asking for these tests. With many physicians, you may need to be your own health advocate. Many new patients at the Center for Health and Wellness who had no obvious signs of heart disease learned that they had hidden cardiovascular problems as a result of more specific testing, sometimes after their standard cardiology evaluations gave them a clean bill of health. Equally important, many people were aware that they had heart disease, but they had been told by their doctors that there was nothing they could do to prevent recurrences.

You Can Prevent Heart Disease and Strokes

Traditional doctors didn't know what to do with Edward N. His story baffled the experts. He first came to the Center for Health and Wellness about 10 years ago walking with a cane and slurring his speech after suffering two strokes. That's not unusual; 50 percent of stroke sufferers have a repeat stroke within a couple of years. What was unusual was that Ed had a stroke at all. He had none of the traditional risk factors.

Ed didn't smoke or drink alcohol, and his cholesterol was quite low at 150. At 155 pounds, he was not overweight. In fact, he appeared quite lean, trim, and muscular. He had big "Popeye-like" forearms from his work as a lifetime roofer, and he was only 48 years old.

Ed's first stroke came without warning. He was driving home from work when he suddenly felt dizzy and had trouble remembering how to drive his truck. He made it home, but found he couldn't speak. His wife drove him to the emergency room where an MRI on his brain detected a blood clot blocking an artery that supplied an area in the side of his brain used for language.

Strokes are lesions in the anatomy of the brain. During a stroke, an area of the brain dies from lack of oxygen. You can tell what area of the brain was affected by the difficulties the stroke survivor develops. Ed had *expressive aphasia*. He could understand language when he heard it, but he couldn't speak. A year after his first stroke, Ed still suffered episodes when he couldn't think of the proper word for simple things, but he had regained much of his ability to communicate.

Ed's second stroke was more devastating, as is usually the case. This time the blood clot affected an area in the back of his brain that controls coordination and balance. After months of physical therapy, he could walk again, but he was noticeably shaky. His doctor told him he would never be able to climb a ladder again. Each expert Ed went to said they could find no reason for his two strokes, and Ed accepted that.

The reason Ed went outside of his HMO to come to the Center for Health and Wellness was something else his doctors told him. They told him that statistically he had an 80 percent likelihood of having a third stroke and those are always worse.

Ed was pleased to learn that the approach of the Wellness Center was different. He was asked questions that might expose risk factors his doctors had missed. Center staff told him they would check new markers in his blood for the answer to why he was having strokes.

When his lab results came back, an answer was immediately obvious. One number jumped out; Ed's homocysteine level was 26, the highest ever seen at the Center for Health and Wellness. Homocysteine is the best single risk factor for stroke. In one study of people who had had a stroke but had no other risk factors, 90 percent had elevated homocysteine. Yet, incredibly, no one ever checked Ed's homocysteine level. This is not an exception. Of all the Center's cardiac patients, only a handful had homocysteine levels checked before they arrive.

Tests to Give You Options Now

When people learn about cases like Ed's, they always ask, "Well, if that's true, why don't other doctors check homocysteine, too?" There's no explanation of why other doctors omit certain steps and measures, but it happens frequently.

Perhaps this woman's story can give us some insight. A 66-year-old woman came to the Center for Health and Wellness from New York after she had suffered a stroke. Like Ed, her doctors told her "there was no reason" for her stroke. She was not overweight, she did not smoke, and she had low cholesterol. (Her doctors told her to take a cholesterol-lowering drug anyway.) After she was seen and her records reviewed, she was told that some other things in her blood could be checked that hadn't been measured before, including her homocysteine.

She told her neurologist of this plan and he asked her, "Why are they checking for homocysteine? Even if it is elevated, there is no drug to lower it." It would appear that from this neurologist's point of view, no drug equals no solution.

The simple truth is that no drug is necessary! It is easy to lower homocysteine quite effectively and reliably with safe and inexpensive nutritional supplements available at your grocery store.

Effective Blood Tests for Cardiovascular Health

There are many similar examples where physicians ignore certain treatment options because "we don't have a drug for it." It seems that doctors automatically use blood measurements to determine what drugs to prescribe. Most ignore nutrient measurements all together. A fundamental shift in the way traditional physicians view the purpose of laboratory measurements may be necessary before they can use nutritional diagnoses and nutritional solutions to help patients achieve and maintain health.

You can learn a lot about your heart and blood vessels by examining your blood. The following five blood tests paint a precise picture of your cardiovascular health:

- Homocysteine
- C-reactive protein
- CoQ10
- Insulin
- VAP cholesterol

Abnormalities in these tests are linked to heart disease and you can use them to detect heart problems you didn't know you had. But they also do something more – they assess your heart health. Each of the tests provides a piece of the puzzle. Taken together, these tests provide an excellent measure of how healthy your cardiovascular system is. You can then use these tests to take action to move away from disease and toward outstanding heart health, vigor, and vitality.

Lower Homocysteine Naturally

Homocysteine was the undiscovered culprit in Edward N.'s history that caused his strokes. Most patients and many doctors have never heard of homocysteine. To find out more about this unknown sinister killer, let's take a look at a process called oxidation.

Oxidation is the process that generates energy. There are examples of oxidation all around you. In physics, fire is rapid oxidation, while rust is a form of slow oxidation. In biology, oxidation is the "slow burn" of metabolism – the process of burning energy to fuel all of your body's work. But just like outside your body, burning inside your body has consequences. If left unchecked, it inflames and damages surrounding tissues. Luckily, nature has a solution.

You are born with extensive "antioxidant systems" that prevent the fire of oxidation from spreading or damaging delicate surrounding structures. You've probably heard of many of these antioxidants, such as vitamin C, vitamin E, carotenoids, and coenzyme Q10.

Homocysteine is an amino acid that your body produces naturally during normal metabolism. It is the final common product of oxidation in your body. This is important because it distinguishes homocysteine from all other risk assessments. Because it accumulates during oxidation, its measurement is a measure of the health of your antioxidant systems.

Antioxidants prevent homocysteine from accumulating in the body. In other words, homocysteine levels indicate how efficient your antioxidant systems are. If your homocycsteine level is high, it means that the fire of oxidation is overwhelming your antioxidants and damaging your heart and blood vessels. Homocysteine is an excellent measure of antioxidant health as well as an actual indicator of cardiovascular inflammation.

At low levels, your body can handle homocysteine, but when the levels inch above the normal range, it damages your arteries. Homocysteine also increases the formation of arterial plaque and makes the platelets in your blood stickier. This increases the risk of forming blood clots, which can cause heart attack, stroke, and pulmonary embolism.

A number of studies demonstrated the link between high homocysteine levels and heart attack and stroke. For example, the Physician's Health Study concluded that participants with high homocysteine levels are three times more likely to have a heart attack.[1]

One of the major causes of elevated homocysteine levels is a deficiency of B vitamins. Additional factors that may increase a person's homocysteine level include:

• Family history of elevated homocysteine
• Age (homocysteine levels rise with age)

- Gender (homocysteine levels are higher in men than women)
- Kidney disease (homocysteine levels rise when the kidneys fail to filter homocysteine adequately)
- Use of medication (homocysteine levels rise with the use of certain drugs, such as phenytoin, methotrexate, cyclosporine, levodopa, theophylline, niacin, and cholestyramine)
- Underactive thyroid gland
- Alcoholism
- Inflammatory bowel disease
- Menopause
- High blood pressure
- Smoking
- Homocysteinuria (a genetic condition in which high levels of homocysteine are excreted in the urine)

Now, the good news: Keeping homocysteine levels in check is quite easy. All you need to do is consume adequate amounts of vitamin B2, vitamin B6, vitamin B12, and folate. The body uses these B vitamins to detoxify homocysteine and turn it into a harmless amino acid. Most adults do not consume sufficient B vitamins in the diet. Recommended doses are 25 milligrams of B2, 25 milligrams of B6, 500 micrograms of B12, and 800 micrograms of folate.

- **Keeping Score:** A simple blood test can assess the amount of homocysteine in your body. An optimal measure is less than 8 mmol/l. (NOTE: You can safely take the recommended vitamin supplements before checking your homocysteine levels.) Want to know more about homocysteine and inflammation? Read chapter 11, Individualizing *Your Doctor's Heart Cure.*

♥ *Maintain a homocysteine level of less than 8 mmol/l.*

Test for C-Reactive Protein (CRP) Annually

C-reactive protein (CRP) is a very effective predictor of heart disease. When the body experiences acute inflammation, injury, or infection anywhere in the body (including the arteries), the liver releases CRP. Normally, the blood contains no CRP. Therefore, its presence indicates a problem somewhere in the body.

Blood tests for C-reactive protein have been around for 30 years, but they have been used as a marker of end-of-life changes when the body begins shutting down before death. Today, the blood tests are far more sensitive and indicate signs of chronic minor inflammation. We can use the ultra-sensitive modern CRP blood tests to detect heart disease. The *British Journal of Urology* published a study that examined the CRP levels of almost 400 people. They found that once the CRP levels reached twice the normal level, their study participants were 150 percent more likely to suffer a heart attack.[2]

Elevated levels of CRP can also indicate potential heart attacks years before they occur. Consider a study in the *New England Journal of Medicine* in 1997, which followed more than 22,000 men as part of the ongoing Physician's Health Study. When the men first enrolled in the study, they were free of heart disease and gave blood samples. Eight years later, 543 of the men experienced a heart attack, stroke, or a blood clot in a major vessel. Researchers compared the blood samples from these men to those from men in the study who did not have cardiovascular disease.

Men with the highest levels of CRP were twice as likely to have had a stroke and three times as likely to have had a heart attack as the men with normal CRP levels. Keep in mind that these elevated CRP levels were present in the blood six to eight years before the cardiovascular event took place.[3]

Other studies found a similar link between CRP and heart attack in women. For example, research at the Brigham and Women's Hospital and Harvard Medical School in Boston demonstrated that CRP is a very strong predictor of future heart attack, even stronger than cholesterol. In one study, women with the highest levels of CRP were at 4.4 times the risk of heart attack as women with the lowest levels.[4]

Elevated CRP levels can also indicate additional medical problems, such as rheumatoid arthritis, rheumatic fever, cancer, tuberculosis, or pneumonia. In addition, CRP can be an excellent tool to assess future cardiovascular problems.

> ♥ *Ask your physician to test your CRP levels each year as part of your annual physical exam.*

• **Keeping Score:** When it comes to C-reactive protein levels, lower is better. Healthy people score below 1 unit; scores above 4 units indicate signs of heart disease. Levels can reach 20 and above as the body approaches death.

> ♥ *Get optimal C-reactive protein of less than 1 unit.*

Optimize CoQ10 Levels Naturally for Heart Health

CoQ10 provides energy for your heart and other major organs. If your heart doesn't have enough CoQ10, it becomes less efficient, which can lead to heart problems including congestive heart failure.

A simple blood test can reveal your CoQ10 level. Most Americans do not get optimal amounts of CoQ10 from their diet. By monitoring your CoQ10 levels, your physician can help you adjust the dose as needed. Read Chapter 9, Give Your Heart Four Nutrients It Needs, to find out more about which supplements to take for optimal heart health.

• **Keeping Score:** Normal values for CoQ10 are 0.8 to 1.5 nanograms per milliliter. Most labs report both a normal range (your CoQ10 level compared to the levels in the population as a whole), as well as therapeutic ranges (the CoQ10 levels thought to help treat disease). Recommended therapeutic CoQ10 level should be between 2.5 to 3.5 ng/ml. There are no known side effects to elevated CoQ10 levels.

> ♥ *Maintain therapeutic levels of CoQ10 from 2.5 to 3.5 ng/ml.*

Monitor Insulin to Prevent Heart Disease

Insulin problems are one of the main causes of heart disease in the United States, and doctors do a poor job of educating their patients about it. Your pancreas releases insulin to regulate glucose (sugar) levels in the blood, which rise after you eat carbohydrates. It also stimulates the storage of triglycerides and proteins. Then insulin signals the cells to absorb glucose from the bloodstream, energizing the cells and controlling the glucose levels in the blood. As soon as you use up your blood sugar, your liver begins releasing stored glucose to maintain a steady supply of energy.

Insulin makes the body more resistant to burning fat. It encourages the body to store extra fat, especially around the middle. It robs the body of energy by slowing the burning of fat for energy. Stated another way, it leaves you fat and tired.

If you have insulin resistance (a condition common among the obese), your tissues become less sensitive to insulin. Your cells do not take up enough glucose, meaning your pancreas must work overtime to produce extra insulin to achieve the same results. Over time, your pancreas becomes fatigued and stops producing enough insulin. This causes your glucose levels to climb abnormally high. When this occurs, you may be diagnosed with Type 2 or adult-onset diabetes. Many people show signs of insulin resistance for some time before their diabetes is diagnosed.

Both genetic and lifestyle factors contribute to insulin resistance and diabetes. The further you get from your ideal weight, the more difficult it is for your body to manage your glucose levels. In addition, lack of exercise contributes to insulin problems. When you exercise regularly, muscle cells can handle insulin and glucose effectively. The less active you are and the less muscle tissue you have, the harder it is for the body to clear glucose from your bloodstream.

Genes also play a role. Diabetes and insulin resistance are more common among Native Americans, Pacific Islanders, and other people of Asian heritage than it is among those of European descent. Genetics is not destiny; most people with a genetic predisposition to insulin resistance can beat the condition by staying lean, exercising regularly, and eating right.

Insulin resistance isn't just a blood sugar problem. It is also linked with a variety of other health concerns, including heart disease, high blood pressure, high levels of triglycerides, and low HDL (good) cholesterol, among others. Few doctors appreciate the importance of insulin in medical problems beyond diabetes.

Doctors can measure your insulin with a simple blood test. It's alarming how few physicians actually do so.

- **Keeping Score:** Most laboratories consider insulin levels in the normal range when they are between 7 and 17 mcU/mL (micro units per milliliter); a healthier score is 10 mcU/ml and below. Many healthy, lean people who exercise regularly have scores under 7 mcU/ml. High levels often indicate diabetes, hypoglycemia, or obesity; lower levels can indicate diabetes as well. If you check your insulin levels regularly, you can detect and manage diabetes in its early stages before it causes cardiovascular damage. If controlling insulin resistance and diabetes is especially important to you, be sure to read chapter 11 carefully.

Keep insulin levels at a healthy level of below 10 mcU/ml.

Detect Most Cholesterol Abnormalities with VAP Cholesterol

It may surprise you to learn that traditional cholesterol scores are very poor indicators of early cardiovascular disease. Many people with high cholesterol never develop heart problems, and at least half of the people who have heart attacks have seemingly normal cholesterol levels.

It's time for a better test, and we now have one: The VAP (Vertical Auto Profile) cholesterol test. In addition to the basic scores (total cholesterol, high-density lipoproteins, low-density lipoproteins, and triglycerides), the VAP test includes new categories of cholesterol measurement. This extra data makes the test much more effective in predicting heart attack or stroke. Even more importantly, the old test only picks up about 45 percent of cholesterol problems, but the VAP test identifies about 90 percent of them.

Using the data from the VAP test, you can determine whether your cholesterol is actually dangerous or if it is present in your bloodstream but virtually harmless in terms of triggering a heart attack. Among the most important new measurements are Lp(a), LDL pattern size, Metabolic Syndrome, and lipid remnants.

• Lp(a) Predicts Heart Attacks

Recent research shows that the size of the cholesterol-carrying particles or lipoproteins in your blood is more important than the amount of cholesterol circulating in your veins. Some types of cholesterol particles tend to stay dissolved in your blood (where they are harmless), while other types settle out and cause cholesterol plaques (which narrow the arteries and cause heart disease). The most dangerous type of lipoprotein is one known as Lp(a).

Researchers found an important (statistical) link between Lp(a) and heart attacks. Research at The University of Pittsburgh indicates that high levels of Lp(a) cholesterol increase heart attack risk by 300 percent! This makes Lp(a) a much better predictor of heart attack than traditional cholesterol tests.

If you have high levels of Lp(a) cholesterol, you may be vulnerable to clogged arteries and heart attack at an early age, especially if your LDL cholesterol is high. Some experts blame elevated levels of Lp(a) for 25 percent of all heart attacks in people under age 60; they claim that 10 to 25 percent of all Americans may have dangerously high levels of Lp(a).

In addition, research shows that smaller lipoprotein particles also cause problems. They tend to be dense and heavy, so they settle into artery-narrowing plaque more easily than larger and lighter particles. The VAP test provides a measurement of particle size as well.

• LDL Pattern Size Identifies Greater Risks

Size also matters when it comes to LDL or the "bad" lipoproteins you've heard about. Once again, the smaller the LDL particles, the greater the risk of heart attack. In fact, studies found that small LDL particles can raise the risk of heart disease by 400 percent.[5]

Ironically, some of the steps doctors prescribe to prevent cardiovascular problems can cause LDL particles to become smaller and more hazardous. For example, medications such as beta blockers and diuretics can cause LDL particles to become small, dense, and dangerous.

• Recognize Metabolic Syndrome with VAP

Metabolic Syndrome is a condition marked by high triglyceride levels, low HDL (good) cholesterol levels, and dangerously small and dense LDL (bad) particles. Unfortunately, traditional doctors rarely diagnose this dangerous constellation of symptoms effectively.

The VAP test readily identifies patients with Metabolic Syndrome because it identifies all of the risk factors with a single blood test. People with Metabolic Syndrome may not yet have life-threatening cardiovascular disease, but the stage is set for trouble unless they take steps to improve their cholesterol profile. (Again, you can lower your cholesterol naturally – you don't have to use drugs in almost all cases. Read chapter 11 to discover how to lower cholesterol naturally.)

• Lipid Remnants Create Plaque Build-up in Arteries

When very low-density lipids (fats) break down, they produce lipid remnants, which contribute directly to plaque buildup in the arteries. Traditional cholesterol tests do not measure remnant levels, and experts consider lipid remnants a risk factor for developing heart disease all by themselves. Fortunately, the VAP test includes measures of this risk factor.

Measuring total cholesterol levels gives you only a partial picture. As Dr. Michael Hennigan, an expert on expanding lipid panel testing writes, "We must know what the multiple variables are and deal with them simultaneously in order to be successful."[6] When it comes to heart health, the more you know, the better.

VAP IDENTIFIES 90 PERCENT OF CHOLESTEROL ABNORMALITIES

The following table compares traditional measures and those using the new VAP method.

Profile	Traditional Test	VAP Test
Total cholesterol	+	+
HDL	+	+
LDL (directly measured)	+	+
Triglycerides	+	+
Non-HDL cholesterol	−	+
Metabolic Syndrome	−	+
Lp(a)	−	+
LDL Pattern Size	−	+
Remnant Lipids	−	+

As the table shows, traditional cholesterol tests often overlook risks when cholesterol levels appear normal. In fact, the old tests pick up only about 45 percent of cholesterol abnormalities, while VAP testing detects about 90 percent of abnormalities.

The VAP is more crucial now with the new cholesterol guidelines set by the National Cholesterol Education Program. The guidelines call for a more aggressive role in diagnosing and treating high cholesterol. The use of VAP can be helpful for early detection of heart disease but the new guidelines may not be. Physicians following the new guidelines will prescribe dangerous cholesterol-lowering drugs for millions more Americans without telling them about the safer alternatives to drug treatment. There are safe and effective treatment options. Most prescription drugs are better reserved for temporary and emergency situations.

Your doctor can order each of these blood tests at the time of your annual physical. If you have any cardiovascular problems, you can repeat the tests twice a year to monitor the condition. The sooner you measure the health of your heart, the sooner you can take steps toward improving any potential problems.

- **Keeping Score:** The data from VAP cholesterol testing isn't reported with a single score but a two to three page report explains your test results.

ARE YOUR LAB RESULTS ACCURATE?

Everyone makes mistakes, even the laboratory technicians handling your medical tests. Some mistakes are easy to spot. For example, when a lab mistakenly reports the testosterone level of a menopausal patient as that of a virile young man, it is logical to suspect something is wrong at the lab. The follow-up test showed a far more reasonable result. Unfortunately, healthcare professionals often fail to detect these errors.

Most errors involve transcription errors. A lab worker may make a mistake transferring information. For the most part, quality control procedures make sure that the laboratory measurements are accurate and reliable most of the time.

There are steps you can take to protect yourself.

- Question lab results that seem unusual. Ask your doctor for a repeat test.
- Compare your lab results with other tests performed at the same time. Most of the time your doctor orders several tests at once. If one test result seems out of line, request a follow-up test.
- Don't make important medical decisions because of a single abnormal test result.

Be wary of any doctor who objects to repeating tests for unusual, abnormal, or dramatically changed results.

Here's another way to double-check your results. When you have lab tests done, also request a common lab test called a Complete Blood Count (CBC). It is a panel of about 25 measurements of the cells in your blood. Many of these measurements involve a detailed analysis of the size, shape, density, and variability of your red blood cells. These parameters provide a virtually unique marker of your blood, and they don't change much over time. If your doctor runs this test with your other blood work, you can be sure that the specimen tested with your name really belongs to you.

Detect Heart Disease Early with Heart Scans

CT scanners allow doctors to get a "picture" of a patient's organs without looking inside. The latest generation of these machines uses Electron Beam Tomography, a machine that delivers a single electron beam at a speed ten times faster than the x-rays used in traditional CT scans. In fact, the electron beam is so fast it can capture images of a human heart as it beats. This noninvasive test is capable of producing images showing calcium deposits and blockages in the arteries.

Doctors can use this test to detect heart disease early. It is painless, and the entire procedure takes only about ten minutes. The process is similar to an x-ray of the body. A radiologist interprets the freeze-framed images to determine the amount of plaque in the arteries.

The test has one limitation: It detects only calcified plaque, not non-calcified or "soft" plaque. A high calcium score on the test predicts the occurrence of cardiac events. In most cases, a suspicious score indicates the need for further testing.

While the blood markers and additional measurements discussed in this chapter provide an excellent indication of the presence of heart disease, a heart scan may be worthwhile in patients who would like to document the actual presence of arterial blockage.

Check This Important Health Measure, Too

In addition to the above blood tests, you can assess an important measure of health on your own - your body composition. Your doctor can also collect these health assessments as part of your routine physical exam every year.

Three Ways to Measure Body Composition

According to the measurements used by most doctors, the Body Mass Index, Arnold Schwarzenegger and Sammy Sosa are obese and Brad Pitt and Michael Jordan are overweight. Doesn't make sense, does it?

As you can see, the widely used Body Mass Index (BMI) can be grossly misleading. The problem is that the BMI uses simple height/weight tables that don't differentiate between muscle and fat. And, since muscle weighs more than fat, a well muscled person will have a higher BMI. Your weight may be fine according to the height-weight tables, but you may be flabby if you don't have much muscle. Or, on the other hand, if you have a lot of muscle, you may fall into the overweight category, even if you are lean and toned.

For a meaningful measure of "fatness," you need to determine the ratio of fat to lean tissues. Of course, you can probably look in a mirror and get a good idea of whether or not you need to lose weight, but it can still be useful to get an objective measure. You can then use that measurement to track your progress.

You can measure body composition in a number of ways. The three most popular are:

- **The skin fold test:** This test involves measuring the thickness of the skin and fat folds at several key spots on your body using a caliper device. The approach is simple, fast, and provides an accurate measure of body fat. You can purchase calipers at exercise equipment stores or online at www.bodytrends.com.
- **Circumference measurement:** This is a crude but useful approximation of body composition based on your waist and hip measurements. All you need to do is measure your waist (at the narrowest point) and your hips (at the widest point), using a tape measure. Your waist should measure at least one inch less than your hips.
- **Electrical impedance:** This technique calculates body fat based on how well your body conducts electricity. (Water-based tissues are good conductors of electricity while fats are insulators.) This approach is not always very accurate, but it can help you assess changes in body composition over time. If you weigh yourself and measure your body fat at the same time of day, you can get a reasonable idea of how your body composition is changing. These electrical impedance scales are widely available at discount stores and often cost less than $100.

There is little point in measuring body composition more than once every two weeks. A healthy range of body fat for men is 10 to 20 percent; for women 15 to 25 percent. In most people, the leaner, the better.

HIP-TO-WAIST RATIO INDICATES HEART ATTACK RISK

Your waist size can help predict whether you are at risk of having a heart attack. A study in the *American Journal of Clinical Nutrition* found that the increased risk begins when your waist is larger than 35 inches if you are a woman or 39 inches if you are a man.

Where on your body you pack on the pounds is also important. "Apples" – people who load up on abdominal or belly fat – are at greater risk of cardiovascular disease than "pears" – those who carry weight on their hips and thighs. In fact, studies show that waist circumference and waist-to-hip ratios are independent risk factors for heart disease. Why? Abdominal fat breaks down more easily into fatty acids that enter the bloodstream and raise harmful triglyceride levels.

If you aren't sure if you are an apple or pear, pick up the tape measure and measure your waist and hips. Divide your waist measurement by your hip measurement. For example, if your hips are 37 inches and your waist is 28 inches, your waist-to-hip ratio is 0.75, which is normal. (You're a pear.) On the other hand, if your hips are 36 inches and your waist is 37 inches, your waist-to-hip ratio is 1.03. (You're an apple.) A healthy waist-to-hip ratio for women is less than 0.8, and for men it is less than 0.95.

Use Your Pulse to Monitor Your Heart's Response

Your heart rate provides an important measure of your cardiovascular health. You can measure your heart rate at any place where you can feel your pulse. Two easy pulse points are the inside wrist and the carotid artery in the neck. Using a stopwatch, count your pulse for ten seconds, then multiply that number by six to get a number of beats per minute.

To Measure Heart-Rate Recovery: Challenge yourself by doing any aerobic exercise (bicycling or using a treadmill, for instance) for five minutes. Without cooling down count your pulse for 10 seconds. Multiply that number by 6 to calculate your per-minute heart rate. Wait two minutes, then calculate your heart rate again. Subtract the second number from the first to see how far your heart rate has dropped.

The average person's heart rate drops by 55 beats (for example, from 180 during peak exercise to 125 two minutes later). People in superior condition may experience a recovery of 70 beats or so. In general terms, the faster you recover from exercise (or the larger the number), the better your overall fitness and the lower your risk of heart disease.

Find the Right Doctor

You owe it to yourself to find a doctor who takes a comprehensive approach to heart disease prevention and treatment. Walk away from doctors who automatically turn to prescription drugs to control your cholesterol. Seek physicians who work with patients to develop exercise programs and who perform tests to assess your cardiovascular health.

Ask friends and relatives about doctors they recommend. If you're moving to a new community, ask your current physician for suggestions in your new locale. Check with your insurance companies to find out if there is a list or panel of participating physicians. If your insurance company works with certain providers, find out about the doctors on that list.

Local medical societies often have physician referral services. Some hospitals also provide names of physicians. Check the yellow pages of your telephone directory under your county's medical society.

Ask These Questions to Find the Doctor You Want

It is appropriate to ask a few questions before choosing the person you want to handle your care. Call and make an appointment to decide whether you are comfortable with the doctor, support staff, and facilities. Do this legwork before you become sick or need immediate care.

Think about the questions you want to ask and write them down before you go. You may not remember them all if you rely on your memory. Consider the following questions:

- Are you accepting new patients?
- Do you accept my insurance plan?
- How long have you been practicing medicine?
- Do you practice alone or are you part of a group?
- What is your attitude about preventative medicine?
- What is your attitude about alternative medicine?
- Do you recommend the use of vitamins and nutritional supplements?
- May I have the names of some of your patients for referrals?

Consider how you feel when you talk to a prospective doctor. Do you feel you can trust this person? Did he or she answer all of your questions satisfactorily? Did you feel at ease with the doctor? Did the doctor have a relaxed "bedside manner"? Did the doctor and staff treat you courteously? You may also want to talk about prospective doctors with other people you know who have a history of cardiovascular problems.

Cultivate a good relationship with your doctor. Open communication is essential for good care. Although you may get information from several sources, it's a good idea to choose one doctor to be your main source. This will be the doctor you feel most comfortable turning to with your concerns.

Don't be shy about taking notes to help you remember everything. You may also consider asking the doctor if you can tape record the conversation to review later. If you don't understand a medical term your doctor mentions, be sure to ask for an explanation. If you don't understand the explanation the first time, be willing to ask a follow-up question to be sure you feel comfortable with the answer.

Footnotes Chapter 5

1 Stamper M et al. A prospective study of plasma homocysteine and the risk of myocardial infarction in US physicians. *Journal of the American Medical Association.* 1992 Aug 19; 268(7):877-881.

2 Mendall M, et al. C-reactive protein and its relation to cardiovascular risk factor. *British Journal of Urology.* 1996; 312:1061-1065.

3 Ridker PM et al. Inflammation, aspirin, and the risk of cardiovascular disease in apparently healthy men. *New England Journal of Medicine.* 1997 Apr 3; 336(14):973-9.

4 Ridker PM et al. C-reactive protein and other markers of inflammation in the rediction of cardiovascular disease in women. *New England Journal of Medicine.* 2000 Mar 23; 342:836-43.

5 Crouse A, et al. *American Journal of Cardiology.* 1995; 23 Suppl B: 53B.

6 Quote from Michael Hennigan, M.D. Expanded Lipid Testing for the Diagnosis and Treatment of Coronary Artery Disease, *Atherotech*: 2002; p. 17.

STEP TWO

Your Action Plan for Heart Health

6

Enjoy Real Food Again

I f you want to live a longer, healthier, and happier life, eat all the natural
foods you love, including steak, omelets, salmon, and lobster. Yes, you
can become lean and healthy – and improve your cholesterol profile, lower
your blood pressure, reverse your diabetes, and lower your heart attack risk
– while eating these fabulous foods.

The Doctor's Heart Cure's basic philosophy of eating is this: Eat foods
that you enjoy in their natural, unadulterated forms. You can eat red meat,
fish, poultry, dairy, eggs, most vegetables, most fruits, berries, and nuts. For
a healthy heart avoid such man-made foods as Twinkies, French fries, artificial cheese spread, processed meats, and Wonder bread. It's just that easy.
By the time you complete this chapter, you'll have identified the wide
variety of natural foods you can include in your heart-healthy diet.

Start with the Real Food Groups

Remember those four basic food groups from grade school health class?
If you've forgotten them, don't worry about it, they don't tell you anything
about your natural diet. They were a nutritionist's attempt to make sense of
a very contrived artificial diet based on grains and other processed foods.

It's simpler and much more consequential to think about your food
according to the macronutrients it contains. A macronutrient is a nutrient
that you burn for energy. There are three basic types: Proteins, fats, and

carbohydrates. This is true if you are talking about the diet of modern Americans, ancient cave dwellers, or space station astronauts. Macronutrients are different chemically and structurally, and each has a different function and a different hormonal response. The type of macronutrients you eat affects your metabolism, *regardless of the number of calories you consume.*

When you eat protein, your body produces growth hormones that build muscles. When you eat carbohydrates, your body secretes insulin to digest carbohydrates and build fat. (Eating fat has little effect on hormone balance.) The effect of eating protein and carbohydrate has a "compounding effect" over time. The body muscle or body fat that you build in response to protein or carbohydrate in your diet then further affects your metabolism. For instance, muscle stimulates testosterone and energy use, while fat stimulates estrogen and energy conservation.

Creating a lean physique at the same time you sidestep this modern epidemic of heart disease is easier than you may think. You create both a lean body and a healthy heart by choosing the right quantity and quality of proteins and carbohydrates. For those of us who eat the typical American diet, this means increasing protein, decreasing carbohydrates, and replacing bad fats with healthy fats.

Simply return to the mix of these macronutrients in your natural diet. This approach will lay the foundation for you to establish the weight and health you were born to enjoy. You also will enhance your energy and strength while losing body fat. Once you try this approach to eating, you'll agree that it's more enjoyable and easier to follow than the American Heart Association's low-fat approach.

Three Easy Principles for Healthy Eating

You don't have to count calories or record fat grams to achieve your ideal weight and maintain optimal cardiovascular health. All you have to do is to eat the same ratio and quality of proteins, fats, and carbohydrates that we have for eons. How are you going to do that? Get started by remembering these three easy principles:

- **Principle #1:** Eat protein at every meal.
- **Principle #2:** Limit carbohydrate intake.
- **Principle #3:** Eat natural fats.

The more you follow these three basic principles, the faster you'll achieve the health and weight you want.

TREAT YOURSELF TO THESE TOP 7 HEALTH BENEFITS

Follow *The Doctor's Heart Cure's* dietary recommendations to enjoy these benefits for you and your family:

(1) **Achieve healthy weight.**

(2) **Enhance your heart health.**

(3) **Improve your cholesterol profile.** A recent study of lean meat and cholesterol proves that people who introduce lean meat into their diet reduce their cholesterol levels. By the way, it doesn't matter whether it is white meat or red meat. Research shows that this lowers bad LDL cholesterol and raises good HDL cholesterol.[1]

(4) **Reduce your risk of heart attack by limiting refined sugar.** A startling study in the *The Lancet* proves the ill effects of refined sugar. The study shows that someone eating 4 ounces of sugar daily is five times more likely to have a heart attack than someone who eats 2 ounces of sugar daily. The average American eats 5 ounces of sugar daily.[2]

(5) **Reduce your risk of developing diabetes.** Many studies prove that low-carbohydrate diets minimize the effects of diabetes. One important study analyzed diabetic patients for 8 weeks. Some of the patients ate a diet with 55 percent of calories from carbohydrates (very similar to the average American's diet). The other group ate a diet with 25 percent of the calories came from carbohydrates. The group eating the 25 percent diet expe-

rienced a significant drop in blood sugar levels, while those eating the 55 percent carbohydrate diet experienced a rise in blood sugar levels. People with diabetes who eat more carbohydrates make their diabetes worse.[3]

(6) **Strengthen your immune system by eating a high-protein diet.** A German study in the *Journal of Nutrition* proves the importance of eating more protein foods. The researchers found that high protein diets boost antioxidant levels. The more protein people eat, the higher their antioxidant levels become. Low protein consumption actually seems to cause damaging oxidative effects of free radicals.[4]

(7) **Avoid certain cancers.** An alarming report out of Stockholm University raises even more concern about processed carbohydrates. The report, released through Sweden's National Food Administration in April 2002, found cancer-causing agents in breads, rice, potatoes, and cereals. Starch transforms into a compound called acrylamide when heated. The US Environmental Protection Agency recognizes acrylamide as a deadly carcinogen.[5] Eating a high-carbohydrate diet may contribute to certain cancers.

Principle #1: Eat Protein at Every Meal

Protein is the only one of the three macronutrients that your body needs each day. High-quality protein is the key to good nutrition and health. Eating more protein than your body needs to meet its daily demands sends the signal "the hunting is good," which causes the body to burn more carbohydrates for energy. When your body doesn't get adequate protein, the body receives the signal the "food is scarce," prompting the body to stockpile calories as body fat to use when times are tough.

Fish, lean meats, eggs, cheese, organic milk, beans, and nuts are all good sources of protein. Eat as much of these foods as you like. You can eat these foods until you are full but you must choose these foods in their natural forms. Follow these guidelines for selecting natural, unadulterated sources of quality protein.

- **Choose "free-farmed" meat and poultry.** Look for "free-farmed" on meat, dairy, and eggs. Free-farmed products remain on pasture from birth to market. Cattle raised this way consume a natural diet of grasses and legumes of their choosing.

The terms "free-roaming" and "hormone free" often lead to misunderstanding. "Hormone free" and "antibiotic free" only guarantee that the meat or poultry product had undetectable levels of hormones and antibiotics at the time of slaughter or processing. This claim does not mean that the grower never injected the animal or fed it hormones or antibiotics throughout its life.

The term "free range" means an animal had daily access to the outdoors for a period determined by the manufacturer. Food producers can make this claim if they opened a door to the outside for just a few minutes a day, whether or not an animal went outside to roam the range.

Most commercial growers fatten their cattle as quickly as possible by feeding them cheap grain and "feedstuff." This can include an unsavory combination of grain, pesticides, hormones, antibiotics, cement dust, candy, animal manure, cardboards, nut shells, feathers, and meat scraps.[6] No kidding.

Not surprisingly, studies have found that the more grass cattle ate, the more nutritious their beef became.[7] If you can't find free-farmed foods in your local supermarket, buy them from a private farmer. You can find a comprehensive list of farmers at www.eatwild.com.

PROTECT YOURSELF FROM THE THREAT OF MAD COW DISEASE

"Mad Cow Disease" is incurable and 100 percent fatal, but it is preventable. Modern animal husbandry created conditions that allowed the spread of Bovine Spongiform Encephalopathy (BSE), better known as Mad Cow Disease. Humans contract the disease when they eat infected beef. The disease has killed 143 people in Great Britain and 10 more elsewhere.

When Mad Cow Disease spread through Europe, US Health officials insisted that it could not come to the United States. When the disease reached Canada in May 2003, The US Food and Drug Administration again offered reassuring words, but the government failed to back up its safe-food claims with policies that would offer meaningful protections.

In nature, cows eat plants, not meat. Cows are infected with BSE when food processors mix the flesh of dead cows with animal feed. Laws currently prohibit the practice of feeding cows to cows. Although unsavory and unnatural, it is legal for food producers to feed cow remains to chickens, and then feed those same chickens back to the cows.

Protect yourself and enjoy the benefits of beef by choosing only grass-fed cattle. Grass-fed beef is an excellent source of protein. (The only food considered a better source of protein is the egg.) When you eat grass-fed beef, you are also getting more B vitamins, CoQ10, and a more favorable ratio of Omega-6 and Omega-3 fatty acids. Plus, grass-fed cattle, is completely free of Mad Cow Disease.

ORGANIC: WHAT THE LABELS REALLY MEAN

Choose organic foods whenever you can. Read the labels and know what the US Department of Agriculture's various organic labels really mean:

Organic: The 'organic' labels on meat, poultry, eggs, and dairy products means food producers fed the animals organic feed, and did not give the animals antibiotics or growth hormones. Additionally, the food producers did not use most conventional pesticides, petroleum-based or sewage-based fertilizers, genetically modified ingredients, or irradiation.

That may seem clear but advertisers, understandably, only want to provide the most favorable features of their product. A little knowledge on your part can allow you to "read through" the labeling to know the facts of what you're considering eating. These are the various USDA categories for organic foods.

- **100 percent organic:** These foods contain only organically produced ingredients. The products must carry the contact information for a USDA-regulated certifying agent; they may carry the "USDA Organic" seal.
- **Organic:** These foods are made from at least 95 percent organic ingredients (the remaining 5 percent must be on a national list of accepted ingredients). The products must list the contact information for a USDA-regulated certifying agent; they may also carry the "USDA Organic" seal.
- **Made with organic ingredients:** These foods consist of at least 70 percent organic ingredients. They must carry the contact information for a USDA-regulated certifying agent; they may not carry the "USDA Organic" seal.
- Food with less than 70 percent organic ingredients may include any organic ingredients in the ingredients list only. These packages may not carry the "USDA Organic" seal or any identifying information for a USDA-regulated certifying agent.

Protein in Common Foods

Beef	7 grams per ounce
Poultry	7 grams per ounce
Fish	7 grams per ounce
Large egg	7 grams per egg
Milk	8 grams per cup
Cheese	7 grams per ounce
Bread	4 grams per slice
Cereal	4 grams per 1/2 cup
Vegetables	2 grams per 1/2 cup
Soybeans (dry)	10 grams per ounce
Peanuts	7 grams per ounce
Lentils (dry)	6.5 grams per ounce
Red beans	6 grams per ounce
Baked potato	9 grams per 8 ounces
Cashews	5 grams per ounce

- **Eat wild fish and seafood.** You may see conflicting information about whether seafood is safe and if it improves cardiovascular health. Research will continue to produce seemingly different answers to this question because it depends on the seafood.

  We know that many types of seafood contain mercury from industrial pollutants. We know that high enough levels of mercury are powerfully toxic to the nervous and circulatory systems of animals and humans. But can we show that current mercury levels in humans actually effect their heart health?

  In a recent Johns Hopkins study, researchers analyzed toenail clippings from about 1400 men, half of whom recently had heart attacks. Mercury levels were 15 percent higher in men who had heart attacks, indicating that higher mercury levels are associated with increased rates of heart attacks.

  Seafood, however, is such an excellent source of high quality protein (third after eggs and red meat) and other nutrients that it is worth searching for safe varieties. Fish is one of the best sources of omega-3 fatty acids, and many studies show that Omega-3 fats keep the heart healthy.

The bottom line? While scientists continue to learn more about mercury's effect on the heart, stay away from fish with the highest amounts of mercury. As a general rule, the larger the fish, the higher up the food chain it is and the more likely it will contain mercury. In other words, dine on small fish rather than large ones, and reserve eating large apex predators for rare occasions. When reviewing the menu, limit your selection of swordfish, tilefish, tuna, and shark, and opt for Pollock, trout, flounder, and salmon, or the very small fish like anchovies and sardines, which tend to have low levels of mercury.

One of the very best fish to eat is wild salmon, especially Alaskan salmon. It has very low levels of mercury, high levels of Omega-3 fatty acids, and is one of the few fish with the vital heart nutrient, CoQ10. Avoid farm-raised or Atlantic salmon, which contain higher levels of mercury and PCBs (pesticides) than wild varieties.

If you catch fish yourself, you can check with local fish advisories. You may also check the Environmental Protection Agency website at www.epa.gov for lists of safe freshwater fish in local areas.

It's also important to prepare fish in a way that preserves their heart-healthy Omega-3 fats. A recent study in Circulation followed 4,000 participants monitoring their heart health for nine years. Those who ate fried fish failed to reap any of the heart-protection benefits normally association with fish consumption.[8] This applies to the fish sandwich at the drive-through. Instead of choosing fried, chose fish prepared by broiling, baking, or grilling.

- **If you're a vegetarian, start to think about eating meat again.** Studies found that 78 percent of all vegetarians on a vegan diet have sky-high homocysteine levels and are deficient in Vitamin B12, putting them at risk of sudden heart death.[9] Researchers compared homocysteine levels in vegetarians, vegans, and omnivores. (The "vegetarians" ate dairy and eggs but no meat, chicken, or fish; vegans eat no animal products of any kind; omnivores eat anything they like.) Compared to the omnivorous group, homocysteine levels were greater than 50 percent higher in the vegan group.

The vegetarians had additional deficiencies as well. Vegans and vegetarians did not consume adequate amounts of the essential amino acid methionine, due to the lower methionine content in plant proteins versus animal proteins. Since vitamin B12 doesn't occur in plants and it is essential to the human diet, all vegetarians that do not effectively supplement suffer from low levels of vitamin B12. In this study, vitamin B12 levels were low enough to be clinically deficient in 78 percent of the vegans, 26 percent of the vegetarians, but none of the omnivores.

The news gets worse. Vegetarians tend to develop severe deficiencies of Coenzyme Q10. CoQ10 is probably the most important single nutrient for your heart, as you'll discover in chapter 8, Energize your Heart: The Miracle of Coenzyme Q10. It provides high-energy output for your heart and brain, and protects them from damage from oxidation. The best source is red meat, especially wild game and organ meat. Of the thousands of patients seen at the Center for Health and Wellness, vegans have the very lowest levels of CoQ10.

- **Drink Your Milk.** There are some who believe that dairy consumption causes a growing list of modern day maladies, from high blood pressure to arthritis. If you cannot digest the carbohydrate lactose, you know to avoid dairy. For the majority though, dairy can provide protein which may outweigh other concerns. A 10-year Harvard Medical School study shows that regular consumption of dairy products lowers the risk of heart disease and type II diabetes. The researchers conclude, "milk is a good source of protein, and may help to prevent serious health problems."[10]

  In another study, scientists compared a group of men who drank milk with a group of men who drank an equal amount of a carbohydrate "performance" drink. Both groups lifted weights for 10 weeks. In the end, the milk group gained more muscle.[11] Before we had performance-enhancing sports drinks and non-dairy, low-fat, soy protein powder shakes, we had old-fashioned milk. Once again, researchers have found that natural is better.

When you buy milk and other dairy products, look for the "organic" label. Harmful animal husbandry practices compromise the potential quality of processed milk. Processed milk tends to be contaminated with unhealthy antibiotics and hormones, and it has the wrong balance of Omega-3 and Omega-6 fatty acids. Spend a few cents more and buy organic dairy products; your health is one of the best investments you'll ever make. Raw, unpasteurized milk is even better if you have access to a farm.

- **Eat nuts.** Several studies show that those who eat nuts are less likely to die from heart disease than those who don't eat nuts. One study in the *Archives of Internal Medicine,* a 17-year review of over 21,000 men, shows that nut eaters are 50 percent less likely to die from heart rhythm problems and 30 percent less likely to die from heart disease than non-nut eaters are. Men who ate about an ounce of nuts twice a week show the most favorable results. The Omega-3 fatty acids in the nuts may protect the heart.

  The US Food and Drug Administration now allows nut manufacturers to tout the health benefits of nuts on their labels. Walnuts, pecans, pistachios, almonds, and hazelnuts earned bragging rights for their package labels.

  Don't look for health benefits from peanuts. Peanuts aren't real nuts; they don't grow on trees. Peanuts are similar to potatoes in that they are both tubers that grow underground. In addition, peanuts don't have the heart healthy Omega-3 fats of nuts.

  Avoid nuts that contain processed ingredients, such sugar coatings, artificial colors, and preservatives. Lastly, check the label for the type of oil used to process the nuts. Many manufacturers cook nuts in peanut oil, which is inflammatory. Look for nuts prepared with safflower, sesame or no oil instead.

PROTEIN IS GOOD FOR YOUR BONES

Many have attacked high protein diets under the mistaken notion that they decrease bone density. Lower bone density is an "associated factor" in developed countries but not caused by protein intake. That false belief fails to account for the very high protein intake and strong bones world-wide prehistoric peoples and modern hunter-gatherers. Now a new, 3-year study of 342 people over the age of 65 found high-protein diets actually help prevent and reverse bone loss.

According to a study in the *American Journal of Clinical Nutrition*, people who had adequate calcium and high protein intakes had the highest bone densities. The researchers conclude that protein helps the body absorb calcium, which in turn negates the adverse affects protein may have on calcium loss from the bones. For strong bones and a healthy heart, eat your protein.

Principle #2: Limit Carbohydrate Intake

Processed carbohydrates, especially starchy ones, make you fat and diseased. Get your carbs from unprocessed vegetables that grow above ground and skip the grains and potatoes.

- **Eat low-glycemic foods.** What makes one food "better" for you than another? Different foods contain different nutrients, of course, but the body handles them differently. For example, all carbohydrates contain four calories per gram, but they can have wildly different effects on the body's blood sugar levels.

Photosynthesis in plants builds carbohydrates. There are several forms:

- Simple sugars (such as honey, fruit sugar and table sugar)
- Starches or complex carbohydrates (including vegetables, such as carrots, potatoes, and yams; and whole grains, such as rice, corn, and wheat)

- Fiber (cellulose or hemicellulose, the indigestible roughage found in unprocessed carbohydrate-containing foods)

The body converts all digestible carbohydrates into glucose or blood sugar. Then the pancreas kicks into gear, producing insulin to move the blood sugar into the cells to use for energy. The body stores any excess as glycogen in the liver and muscles or as body fat.

Recent studies have found a link between processed starches and heart attack. All grains must be processed before we humans can eat them. Many studies, including a recent one from Spain, link processed starches to heart attacks.[12] These processed starches can come from lasagna, bread, cookies, spaghetti, pizza, crackers, chips, and cereals. These foods cause an unnatural surge in blood sugar. Your body responds by secreting excessive insulin until your blood sugar returns to normal. Because there is so much glucose tightly packed into these starches, your body secretes more insulin for a longer time than if you ate sources of simple sugars such as fruit. This prolonged and excessive release of insulin makes us fat, and it causes heart disease.

Carbohydrates vary in how high and fast they raise blood sugar levels. The higher the blood sugar level and the faster the rise, the higher the glycemic index score. Researchers calculate the glycemic index by feeding 100 grams of the food in question to a volunteer and measuring his or her blood sugar every half an hour. They then compare these numbers to the blood sugar produced by ingesting the same amount of glucose solution (sugar water). For example, a peach has a glycemic index of 40. That means that it produces a blood sugar level that is 40 percent of the blood sugar level produced by drinking the same amount of sugar water.

The lower the glycemic index, the less impact a food will have on your blood sugar. You can use the "glycemic index" to help you make wise food choices.

- **The Glycemic Index** The following chart assigns a glycemic index score to common carbohydrates based on how much the food spikes blood sugar levels. The list is a sampling of foods tested in a clinical setting.

The Glycemic Index

Food	GI Score	Food	GI Score
BAKED GOODS		**CEREAL**	
Corn bread	110	Kellogg's Corn Flakes	92
French bread	95	Kellogg's Crispix	87
Donut	76	Corn Chex	83
Waffle	76	Kellogg's Rice Krispies	82
Graham cracker	74	Corn Pops	80
Kaiser roll	73	Grapenuts	75
Bagel	72	Kellogg's Bran Flakes	74
Melba toast	70	Cheerios	74
White bread	70	Kellogg's Special K	69
Corn tortilla	70	Quaker Oats Life	66
Whole wheat bread	70	Muselix	66
Taco shell	68	Quick Oats Inst. Porridge	65
Angel food cake	67	Kellogg's Raisin Bran	61
Croissant	67		
Stoned wheat thins	67	**DAIRY**	
Flan cake	65	Ice cream (reduced fat)	47
100% whole rye bread	65	Pudding	44
Rye crisps	65	Milk (whole)	40
Bran muffin	60	Ice cream	38
Blueberry muffin	59	Yogurt (plain)	36
Whole wheat pita	57		
Oatmeal cookie	55	**VEGETABLES**	
Sara Lee Poundcake	54	Potato	104
Betty Crocker Vanilla		Parsnip	97
cake w/vanilla frosting	42	Carrots	92
Pumpernickel bread	41	Corn (sweet)	60
Betty Crocker Chocolate		Beets (canned)	64
cake w/Chocolate frosting	38	Sweet potato	54
		Yam	51
		Peas	48
BEVERAGES		Tomato	38
Gatorade	78	Artichokes	0
Ocean Spray		Beans (string or green)	0
Cranberry Juice Cocktail	68	Broccoli	0
Coca Cola	63	Cabbage	0
Orange juice	57	Cauliflower	0
Nestle Hot Chocolate Mix	51	Celery	0
Grapefruit juice	48	Eggplant	0
Pineapple juice	46	Mushroom	0
Soy milk (full fat)	44	Peppers	0
Soy milk (low fat)	44	Spinach	0
Apple juice	41	Squash	0
Tomato juice	38		

Sources: Miller, J., et al. The New Glucose Revolution: Marlow & Company, New York, 1996. The Glycemic Index at www.glycemicindex.com. Diabetes Mall at http://www.diabetesnet.com.

The Glycemic Index

Food	GI Score	Food	GI Score
FRUIT		**MEAL REPLACEMENT BARS**	
Watermelon	72	Pure-Protein Bar	
Pineapple	66	(Strawberry shortcake)	43
Cantaloupe	65	Pure-Protein Bar	
Raisins	64	(White chocolate mousse)	40
Apricot (canned in		Pure-Protein bar	
light syrup)	64	(Chocolate Deluxe)	38
Papaya	60	L.E.A.N. Nutribar	
Peaches (can in		(Chocolate Crunch)	32
heavy syrup)	58	L.E.A.N. Nutribar	
Kiwi	58	(Peanut Crunch)	30
Fruit cocktail		Pure-Protein Bar	
(drained, Delmonte)	55	(Chewy chocolate chip)	30
Peaches		Pure-Protein Bar	
(canned in light syrup)	52	(Peanut butter)	22
Banana	51		
Mango	51	**MEAT/PROTEIN**	
Dates (dried)	50	Beef	0
Orange	48	Cheese	0
Pear (canned in pear juice)	44	Chicken	0
Grapes	43	Eggs	0
Apple	40	Fish	0
Strawberries (fresh)	40	Lamb	0
Pear	34	Pork	0
Apricot (dried)	32	Veal	0
Prunes	29		
Peach (raw)	28	**NUTS**	
Grapefruit	25	Almonds	0
Plum	24	Brazil nuts	0
Cherries	22	Hazelnuts	0
		Macadamia	0
		Pecans	0
LEGUMES		Walnuts	0
Baked beans	48	Cashews	22
Black-eyed peas, boiled	42		
Pinto beans, boiled	39		
Butter beans	36	**NUTRITIONAL-SUPPORT**	
Chickpeas, boiled	31	**PRODUCTS**	
Marrowfat peas, boiled	31	Enercal Plus	61
Navy beans, boiled	31	Ensure	50
Lentils	28	Choice DM	23
Kidney beans	23		
Soy beans, boiled	20		
Peanuts	13		

Sources: Miller, J., et al. The New Glucose Revolution: Marlow & Company, New York, 1996. The Glycemic Index at www.glycemicindex.com. Diabetes Mall at http://www.diabetesnet.com.

If you look at groups of foods together and compare their glycemic indexes, you can make surprising discoveries. Notice that glycemic index has little to do with sweetness. Very sweet cherries have a low index of 22, which is less than one third the index of whole wheat bread! Notice that all the highest glycemic foods are products made from grains or tubers (which grow below the ground). The starchiest of all foods, corn bread and potatoes, have glycemic indexes greater than 100, meaning your blood sugar will go higher when you eat these starches than if you drank an equal amount of sugar water. Think of the glycemic index as a measure of starchiness, not sweetness.

One more interesting discovery, fat in a food lowers its glycemic index. Chocolate cake with chocolate icing has one half the index of a low-fat bagel. Since the tendency of a food to make you fat is its glycemic index combined with how much of it you eat, these discoveries are real revelations, and they go a long way to explaining the difficulty with reducing your body fat on a low-fat diet.

This glycemic index may seem complicated, but it all boils down to a few simple guidelines:

- Avoid grains, including "whole grains." Cereals are no more natural to your diet than is the box they're sold in.
- Avoid potatoes and other tubers that grow below ground.
- Eat veggies that grow above the ground.
- Don't eat corn. It is a grain.
- Don't opt for low-fat varieties of processed foods.
- Don't eat foods with added sweeteners.
- Choose high-fiber foods. Fiber slows digestion, so the sugar in fiber-rich foods tends to hit your blood stream slowly.

Principle #3: Eat Natural Fats.

Fat does not spike your blood sugar or insulin. Natural fats are a healthy part of a balanced diet. Get your fat from free-range or grass-fed animals, eggs, nuts and unprocessed vegetable oils. These are some of the healthiest foods you can eat, not health hazards.

The health benefit of natural fats comes from their balance of Omega-3 and Omega-6 fatty acids. Omega-3 fatty acids are a type of polyunsaturated fat that have a favorable effect on the heart. Studies show that Omega-3s prevent irregular heartbeat, reduce arterial plaque, decrease blood clotting, lower blood pressure, and minimize inflammation. Omega-6 fatty acids – found in many processed foods – interfere with the functioning of Omega-3s.

As is often true in nature, balance is essential. Our bodies need both Omega-3s and Omega-6s, but we need them in the right ratios. For most of the time humans have been on Earth, we ate foods containing Omega-6's and Omega-3's in a ratio of about 2:1. However, over the last 75 years in North America, Omega-6's in the diet have soared and now the ratio is 20:1. The average American eats ten times as much Omega-6 as is healthy. The main sources are vegetable oils, processed foods, and grain-fed meat.

That is where the health gurus of the 1980s made another big mistake. They mistook the heart disease culprit to be red meat because Western livestock has an unhealthy Omega-6: Omega-3 fatty acid ratio of 20:1. They never bothered to explain why native people who ate about 85 percent of their calories as wild red meat lacked modern heart disease.

If you measure Omega-6s and Omega-3s in wild range or grass-fed animals, you get a dramatically reversed and heart healthy ratio of 0.16 to 1. Stated another way, the culprit isn't the fat natural to red meat; it's the environment producing the changed fat in modern farmed red meat. It turns out that nature has combined the best source of quality protein with the best source of heart healthy Omega-3 fats – at least when animals are permitted to eat their natural wild diet. If you eat organic meats and avoid processed foods you can restore a more healthful balance of fatty acids.

- Avoid Trans Fats. A generation ago, food manufacturers concocted trans fats through a process called hydrogenation. Trans fats increase shelf life and stabilize foods. But this process also changes the biological function of your essential fatty acids.

  Trans fats lurk in the majority of the processed foods on supermarket shelves – from treats like chocolate-chunk cookies, Krispy Kreme doughnuts, and cheese curls to presumed healthy foods like granola bars, multigrain snack chips, low-fat cookies, and high-fiber breakfast cereals. Worse yet, many foods with trans fats bear labels bragging that they contain low cholesterol or low saturated fat.

Trans fats wreak havoc on cholesterol levels. They raise LDL ("bad") cholesterol and reduce HDL ("good") cholesterol, while at the same time increasing triglycerides. Trans fats also contribute to heart disease. In 2001, the British medical journal *The Lancet* published a comprehensive Dutch study addressing the effects of consuming trans fatty acids. Researchers found that trans fatty acid intake is directly associated with an increased risk of coronary heart disease.

Trans fats have no place in your diet. Food manufacturers add these to your food without your consent. We are unwitting participants in an experiment with our food supply. These harmful trans fats trigger heart disease and additional health problems.

By January 1, 2006, the labels on foods and dietary supplements must contain a line that lists the amount of trans fat in the product. Although some manufacturers already started to include trans fat information, currently there is no requirement that they do so. Trans fats are found in most (but not all) margarines, crackers, cookies, pastry products, snack foods, frozen dinners, breads, some cereals, the oil used for deep-frying in fast-food restaurants and other foods.

Avoid foods that list "hydrogenated" or "partially hydrogenated" vegetable shortening or vegetable oil among the ingredients.

• Avoid all processed low-fat foods. If a package bears a "low-fat" label, avoid it. It is probably bad for your heart. Manufacturers add more carbs to compensate for the loss of taste caused by removal of the fat. And the added carbs are the worse kind of refined, processed carbs – the major cause of heart disease. In a study of 80,000 nurses, Harvard researchers calculate that substituting an equal number of calories of carbohydrates for the polyunsaturated fats increases the risk of heart disease by over 50 percent. Removing the natural fats and adding carbohydrates is bad for your heart.[13]

THE PROBLEM WITH FAST FOOD

The real problem with fast food is not that it has too much fat. The real problems are that it contains man-made trans fats, it's loaded with processed carbs, the fish, chicken, and potatoes are fried in processed oils; and the red meat comes from grain-fed, artificially maintained and fattened animals.

What can you do?

If you want good nutrition in a hurry, the selection at Boston Market has little trans fats or processed carbs, and there are several high-protein choices. If you think you must eat at one of the fast-food chains, here are tips to follow:

- Choose the leanest red meat.
- Choose grilled fish or chicken over fried.
- Skip the trans fat containing salad dressing.
- Throw the bun in the garbage.
- Skip the vegetable oil cooked fries.
- Drink water with your lunch.

If possible, stop by a local supermarket or seafood restaurant. You can pick up a much healthier meal in about the same amount of time.

Say "No" to Genetically Altered Foods

Genetically altered foods are not the stuff of science fiction. These foods are on our grocery store shelves right now. In fact, by the US Department of Agriculture's own estimates, an astounding 70 percent of processed foods sold in the United States contain genetically modified organisms (GMO). You probably eat these foods every day, but you may not know it because the USDA doesn't require food manufacturers to tell you if there are GMOs in your food.

Surprised? You may have thought the USDA requires labeling of genetically modified foods so you could choose if you want to eat them. Not this time.

FlavSavr was the first food producer to introduce genetically modified foods when they produced their "new and improved" tomato in 1994. A biotech company inserted a foreign gene from a fish into the tomato to make it stay fresh longer. Bioengineering spread to strawberries, corn, soybeans, tobacco, wheat, and rice, among other foods. And these ingredients have since made their way into sports drinks, cake mix, baby food, frozen dinners, hamburger buns, cereal, and just about every other food you can imagine.

No Pre-Market Safety Testing for GMO Foods

The United States is one of the only countries that treats genetically altered organisms like natural foods:

- The US has no mandatory pre-market safety testing of GMOs.
- GMOs need not be identified on food labels.
- Official Food and Drug Administration policy does not make a distinction between genetic engineering and breeding.

Here are a few steps you can take to regain some choice in the matter.

- Buy foods labeled "non GMO." Some manufacturers of products that do not contain genetically modified ingredients now label them as "non-GMO."
- Call the manufacturers of your favorite foods and ask if they contain GMOs. Let manufacturers know your position on the issue.
- You can find a comprehensive list of non-GMO and GMO foods at www.truefoodnow.org/gmo facts/product_list/pf-list.html.

Heart Health Benefits for Moderate Drinkers

You've probably heard that drinking moderate amounts of red wine appears to benefit your cardiovascular health. But do other alcoholic beverages offer similar health benefits? Let's look at the evidence.

- **Red wine:** Science has noted the protective polyphenols in red wine for several years. New evidence identifies additional health benefits of wine. A study in the 2001 issue of *Nature* explains that red wine blocks the formation of endothelin-1, a chemical that makes blood vessels constrict and increases heart attack risk. Antioxidants in wine also reduce the formation of plaque in blood vessels. More studies find that wine dilates blood vessels. Still others suggest wine stops blood from inappropriate clotting.

- **Beer:** Researchers at the University of Texas Southwestern Medical Center found that drinking moderate amounts of beer lowered a person's chance of heart disease by 30 to 40 percent compared to non-drinkers. Another study in *The New England Journal of Medicine* in November 1999 found that light to moderate beer-drinking decreases a person's risk of having a stroke by 20 percent.

- Additional research found that the yeast in beer is rich in vitamin B6. Studies link vitamin B6 to heart health. Beer increases vitamin B6 in blood plasma by 30 percent.

- **All alcohol:** Other studies have not discriminated between types of alcoholic beverages people drink. For example, the Physician's Health Study found that men who have 5 to 6 drinks a week have 20 percent lower risk of death than those who don't drink at all. Those who consumed alcohol daily have a 40 percent decrease in the risk of cardiovascular disease. But you can have too much of a good thing. The study also found that men who drink more than two drinks a day have a higher risk of death.

The Cardiovascular Health Study found a similar link between alcohol and stroke. The study, published in a 2001 issue of *Stroke*, followed 3,660 people over age 65 for 2 years. People who drink between one and six alcoholic drinks per week have a lower incidence of stroke and brain abnormalities compared to those who do not drink at all.

Alcohol can also lower your risk of developing diabetes. In a 2001 issue of the medical journal *Diabetes*, researchers reported the results of a 12-year study of 47,000 men from age 40 to 75 that examined the association of alcohol with diabetes. The conclusion: men who drink 1.5 drinks a day have a 36 percent lower risk of developing diabetes. Moderate alcohol intake may improve the sensitivity of insulin and lower blood sugar levels.

If you currently do not drink alcohol, don't start now just to protect your heart. There are more important steps you can take to benefit your cardiovascular health. If you currently drink, do so in moderation. In virtually all of the studies on alcohol use, only moderate drinkers, those who consume one or two drinks per day, tend to benefit.

The Truth About Your Drinking Water

No doubt about it, clean drinking water is vital to good health. Water accounts for 60 percent of your total bodyweight and 75 percent of your muscle tissue. It transports nutrients to your cells and carries away waste.[14] Water is your body's most essential nutrient.

But bottled water is also big business. A generation ago, no one dreamed that Americans would someday pay more for water than they do for gasoline, but we do. The multi-billion, bottled-water industry plays on the public's fears of contamination. Don't buy into the hype. It is possible to get safe water from your tap.

First, remember that water is not naturally "pure."

In the environment, water absorbs or dissolves minerals as it flows in streams, sits in lakes, or filters through layers of rock and soil in the ground. Many of these substances, like the minerals calcium and magnesium, provide nutrients and enhance taste.[15]

Our water purification plants filter many impurities out of our tap water before it reaches the faucet. The US Environmental Protection

Agency monitors municipal water supplied for more than 80 possible contaminants. However, the EPA tests water suppliers, not individual homes. Contamination of water is still possible after it leaves the treatment plant. The greatest risks of contamination faces people who live within five miles of farmlands (due to the risk of pesticide contamination) and those who live in homes built before 1986 (these houses may have lead pipes or solder that can leach lead into your water). If you live in an older home or in an agricultural area, test your tap water.

Don't assume that bottled water is always safer than tap water. Despite federal, state, and industry regulations, contaminants sometimes sneak into bottled water. The Natural Resources Defense Council (NRDC) conducted a four-year study, testing more than 1,000 bottles of 103 brands of bottled water. One third of the waters tested contained contaminants of synthetic organic chemicals, bacteria, and arsenic. Some samples exceeded allowable limits under either state or bottled-water-industry standards.[16] Want to know how well your favorite brand did? View the NRDC's test results at www.nrdc.org/water/drinking/bw/appa.asp.

You can also forget the advice to drink distilled water. Long-term use of distilled water can lead to mineral deficiencies that can cause heart beat irregularities and hair loss.[17] Don't cook with distilled water either; cooking with this mineral-depleted water draws many of the nutrients out of food.

Avoid Plastics

In recent years, experts questioned the safety of water sold in plastic bottles. Evidence suggests that polycarbonate plastic is toxic because it contains Bisphenol A (BPA). A study reported in *Current Biology* found exposure to BPA resulted in birth abnormalities in mice. Although the effect on humans remains unknown, mice and humans have a very similar cell division program for eggs.[18] At this point, there aren't any conclusive studies documenting the safety or toxicity of many plastics. One thing is clear, however, these plastics do not exist in nature. To be on the safe side, if you buy water, buy it in glass bottles.

If you want to improve the safety of your tap water, take the following steps:

- Request a water quality report from your water supplier.
- Test your water. Water kits are available to test for bacteria, lead, pesticides, nitrates, nitrites, chlorine, PH, hardness, and arsenic. Reasonably priced kits are available at www.watersafetestkits.com and www.quickpack.com.
- Let the water run a few seconds after you turn on the tap before filling your water glass.
- If your tap water needs improvement, consider using a carbon-block filter. Look for a filter that removes particles that are less than or equal to one micron in diameter for protection from parasites.

If you want to drink bottled water:

- Choose glass bottles.
- Look on the bottom of the containers for the recycling code. Avoid recycling code #7 for polycarbonates.. Recycling codes #1, #2, and #4 denote polyethylene; #5 indicates polypropylene. Use plastics only when necessary.
- Store bottled water away from sunlight and away from household chemicals.
- Don't reuse bottles. Avoid refilling water bottles to prevent bacteria growth and contamination.

Healthy Cooking: Don't Overdo It

You've made wise food choices. You've come up with delicious and inspiring recipes. Now all you have to do is prepare your food properly. You can still get into trouble if you follow conventional advice!

You've probably heard that meat isn't safe unless you cook it until it's brown. Once again, this advice is dangerously wrong. Overcooking food denatures proteins, breaks down vitamins, and removes nutrients. Still worse, cooking at high temperatures triggers a chemical reaction called glycation.

Glycation binds protein and glucose molecules in the body. It results in a disfigured protein assembly or a glycotoxin. As glycotoxins accumulate in your cells, they send out chemical signals that cause inflammation. In addition, these abnormal proteins do not regenerate; they remain damaged forever. This process contributes to premature aging and disease. Conditions associated with glycation and inflammation include aging, diabetes, cancer, arthritis, cardiovascular disease, and Alzheimer's disease.

When we overcook foods, large amounts of glycotoxins collect in the food. A new study demonstrates that if we eat these foods, the glycotoxins transfer to our tissues. Researchers at the Mt. Sinai School of Medicine evaluated two groups of people who had diabetes. One group ate a diet low in glycotoxins, and the other group ate a diet high in glycotoxins. After only two weeks, the high-glycotoxin group had up to 100 percent more glycotoxins in their blood and urine than those who ate the low-glycotoxin diet.[19] Clearly, glycotoxins transfer from your food into your body.

To make matter worse, overcooking denatures many important nutrients in food. One of the best examples is CoQ10. You need CoQ10 for healthy functioning of all of the major organs in your body. Overcooking meat destroys CoQ10.

To avoid glycation, keep the following tips in mind:

- Cook food at lower heat. Low heat doesn't have to mean low taste. Use plenty of spices and fresh herbs to boost the taste of meals.
- When cooking, rely on steaming, stewing, boiling, poaching, and oven baking. Limit highly fried or charred food to no more than a couple of times a week.
- Marinate your meat. When you broil – and even if you occasionally char food – the moisture from the marinade slows down the process of glycation. (Coincidentally, food usually tastes better when it's juicy.) Some favorite marinades include olive oil, wine, garlic, vinegar, citrus juice, and crushed tomatoes in any combination.
- Take a carnosine supplement. Researchers discovered that supplemental carnosine helps prevent glycation. A recent laboratory study shows that supplemental carnosine plays a role in disposing of glycated proteins in tissues.[20] The recommended dose is 1000 milligrams of carnosine daily to minimize glycation.

Eating Well on a Budget

While you can spend a fortune on prime cuts and seafood delicacies, you don't have to – you can eat well on a budget.

- **Eat eggs.** When I was in college, I nearly lived on eggs, the perfect food. Even if you buy organic eggs at $3.00 a dozen, you are spending only 25 cents an egg, or less than a dollar for a very filling meal of the highest quality protein.
- **Brown-bag it.** Taking your lunch and eating more home-cooked meals is a lot more economical – and better for you – than eating out. If you shop according to the guidelines, you know for sure what you're eating.
- **Snack on fruits and nuts.** Avoid processed and snack foods that can rack up the bucks, calories, starches and trans fats. Nuts make very satisfying and nutritious snacks and an apple, pear or peach makes some of the least expensive snacks.
- **Watch for sales.** There are specials even for organic foods.
- **Buy a simple carbon water filter for your kitchen faucet.** If your tap water tests safe, you can save money from not having to buy bottled water.

Eating well provides you with the energy to live a quality life, helps you achieve and restore your health, and reduces medical bills over the long haul. Enrich your life; invest in good health.

TURN THE USDA PYRAMID UPSIDE DOWN

The US Department of Agriculture's Food Pyramid is a formula for dietary disaster. It recommends that Americans eat 6 to 11 servings of grain products every day. Grains, as described earlier in this chapter, contribute to obesity and heart disease. It's no wonder that according to the National Center for Health Statistics, 61 percent of Americans are now overweight.

The Harvard School of Medicine attempted to update the pyramid by advising only whole grains. This switch is healthier for other reasons, but whole grain bread actually spikes blood sugar levels just as much as white bread. *The International Journal of Obesity* reported a study comparing starches and weight. Subjects who ate a low-starch diet weighed markedly less than those who ate a high-starch diet.[21]

In addition to the excess grains, both pyramids lack effective amounts of healthy protein. Protein is imperative to achieve optimal weight and avoid obesity. A recent article in *Arteriosclerosis, Thrombosis, and Vascular Biology* reported that a high-protein diet decreased the risk of obesity. This study also identified the mechanism that links protein and fat production. The researchers discovered that the high-protein diet increases a substance called PAI-1 in the blood. The scientists believe that PAI-1 then directly inhibits the production of fat.[22]

For these reasons, consider turning the USDA food pyramid on its head. Look at this version of the food pyramid:

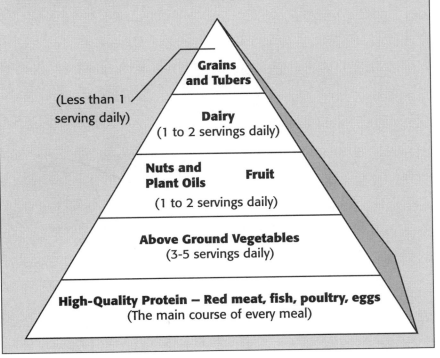

Grains and Tubers
(Less than 1 serving daily)

Dairy
(1 to 2 servings daily)

Nuts and Plant Oils   **Fruit**
(1 to 2 servings daily)

Above Ground Vegetables
(3-5 servings daily)

High-Quality Protein — Red meat, fish, poultry, eggs
(The main course of every meal)

ACTION PLAN

- **Eat quality protein.**
  - Eat protein at every meal.
  - Choose free-farmed meat and poultry.
  - Eat seafood, especially Alaskan or wild salmon.
  - Drink organic milk.

- **Eat quality carbohydrate.**
  - Eat low-glycemic foods. All real vegetables and berries are okay. NOTE: potatoes (tubers) and corn (grain) are not vegetables.
  - Avoid high-glycemic foods. Do not eat grain products (cereals).

- **Eat quality fat.**
  - Increase Omega-3 fats. Good sources of Omega-3s include grass-fed red meat, fish, olives, eggs, nuts, and avocados. NOTE: Peanuts are not true nuts.
  - Decrease Omeage-6 fats.
  - Avoid all trans fats.

- **Avoid problems created by the modern food industry.**
  - Avoid genetically modified foods.
  - Avoid all "low-fat" packaged foods.
  - Do not overcook your foods.

Footnotes Chapter 6

1 Hunninghake DB, Maki KC, Kwiterovich PO Jr, et al. Incorporation of lead red meat into a National Cholesterol Education Program Step I diet: a long-term randomized clinical trial in free-living persons with hypercholesterolemia. *Journal of the American College of Nutrition.* 2000 Jun; 19(3):351-360.

2 Yudkin J. et al. Sugar Consumption and Myocardial Infarction. *Lancet* 1972: 296-297.

3 Gutierrez M, Akhavan M, Jovanovic L and Peterson CM. Utility of a short-term 25% carbohydrate diet on imiproving glycemic control in type 2 diabetes mellitus. *Journal of the American College of Nutrition.* 1998 Dec; 17(6):595-600.

4 Deming DM, Boileau AC, Lee CM and Erdman JW Jr. Amount of dietary fat and type of soluble fiber independently modulate postabsorptive conversion of beta-carotene to vitamin A in Mongolian gerbils. *Journal of Nutrition.* 2000 Nov; 130(11): 2789-2796.

5 "Swedish Scientists Find Cancer Agent in Staple Foods." *Reuters News*: April 23, 2002.

6 Robinson J. *Why Grassfed is Best.* Vashon Island Press: WA 2000, pg. 10.

7 French P, Stanton C, Lawless F, et al. Fatty acid composition, including conjugated linoleic acid, of intramuscular fat from steers offered grazed grass, grass silage, or concentrate-based diets. *Journal of Animal Science.* 2000 Nov; 78(11):2849-2855.

8 Mozaffarin D, Lemaitre RN, Juller LH, et al. Cardiac benefits of fish consumption may depend on the type of fish meal consumed: the Cardiovascular Health Study. *Circulation.* 2003 Mar 18; 107(10):1372-1377.

9 Kanauchi M, Tsujimoto N and Hashimoto T. Advanced glycation end products in nondiabetic patients with coronary artery disease. *Diabetes Care.* 2001 Sep; 24(9):1620-1623.

10 Pereira MA, Jacobs Dr Jr, Van Horn L, et al. Dairy consumption, obesity, and the insulin resistance syndrome in young adults: the CARDIA Study. *Journal of the American Medical Association.* 2002 Apr 24; 287(16): 2081-2089.

11 Puglisi J., et. Al. *Med Sci Sports Exercise*, ASCM Conference, 2002, #2789.

12 Serra-Majem L, Ribas L, Tresserras R, et al. How could changes in diet explain changes in coronary heart disease? The Spanish paradox. *American Journal of Clinical Nutrition*. 1995 Jun; 61(6 Suppl):1351S-1359S.

13 Stampfer MJ, Hu FB, Mansen JE, et al. Primary prevention of coronary heart disease in women through diet and lifestyle. *New England Journal of Medicine*. 2000 Jul 6; 343(1):16-22.

14 Boyle MA. *Personal Nutrition*, fourth Ed., Wadsworth 2001; p. 202.

15 US Environmental Protection Agency, http://www.epa.gov/safewater/dwh/contams.htm

16 Natural Resources Defense Council, www.nrdc.org/water/drinking'nbw.asp.

17 Day C. "Why I Say No to Distilled Water Only," Health and Beyond Weekly Newsletter, reprinted at http://www.mercola.com/article/Diet/water/distilled_water_2.htm.

18 Hunt PA, Hunt KE, Susiarjo M, et al. Bisphenol a exposure causes meiotic aneuploidy in the female mouse. *Current Biology*. 2003 Apr 1; 13(7):546-553.

19 Vlassara H, Cai W, Crandall J, et al. Inflammatory mediators are induced by dietary glycotoxins, a major risk factor for diabetic angiopathy. *Proceedings of the National Academy of Science USA*. 2002 Nov 26; 99(24)15596-15601. Erratum in 2003 Jan 21; 100(2):763.

20 Yeargans G and Seidler NW. Carnosine promotes the heat denaturation of glycated protein, *Biochemical Biophysical Research Communications*. 2003 Jan 3; 300(1):75-80.

21 Rabast U, Schonborn J and Kasper H. Dietetic treatment of obesity with low and high carbohydrate diets: comparative studies and clinical results. *International Journal of Obesity*. 1979; 3(3):201-211.

22 Lijnen R, Marquoi E, Morange P, et al. Nutritionally induced obesity is attenuated in transgenic mice overexpressing plasminogen activator inhibitor-1. *Arteriosclerosis, Thrombosis and Vascular Biology*. 2003 Jan 1; 23(1):78-84.

7

Build a Strong Heart:
Get More For Less

I t's time to re-condition your heart and lungs. First, you need to forget most of what you've heard about "cardio" exercise. Many experts *falsely* believe that to strengthen your heart you must spend hours in the gym each week, pounding out the miles on the treadmill or spinning your wheels on an exercise bike. This classic cardiovascular exercise prescription doesn't work to strengthen your heart, and it causes other problems.

You can transform your heart health following a different approach that takes as little as 10 minutes a day. The rationale behind this different approach to exercise was explained in Chapter 2, Sidestep the "Cardio" Exercise Myth. This chapter provides you with a step-by-step plan to put *The Doctor's Heart Cure's* exercise program into action.

Hundreds of patients at the Center for Health and Wellness have helped develop this uniquely effective fitness program while building their heart capacity and functional strength. If they can do it, you can, too. And in a few short weeks, you'll begin to see and feel the results.

PACE™ *for Cardiovascular Fitness*

<u>P</u>rogressively <u>A</u>ccelerating <u>C</u>ardiopulmonary <u>E</u>xertion™ or **PACE™** – will gradually challenge your heart, lungs, and blood vessels to build their strength. ("Cardio" means heart and "pulmonary" means lungs.) To accomplish this, you will do a series of short bursts of exercise with periods of rest in between. As you get used to these brief challenges you will gradually increase their intensity.

Here are several key concepts to keep in mind as you proceed:

Progressively

Progressively means doing a little bit more this week than you did the week before. Pushing just a little bit harder with each exercise session causes your level of fitness to improve over time. You can add resistance or pick up the pace. Gradually increasing the magnitude of the challenge (rather than the length of the challenge) will coach your body into building greater heart and lung capacity to meet any unexpected challenges you may encounter.

Accelerating

Accelerating refers to training your body to respond to exercise faster. When you are out of condition, it takes several minutes to get your breathing and heart rates up. As your physical condition improves your body gears up for exercise more easily. As your body adapts better, you exploit this capacity to gear up faster by increasing the challenge quicker.

You will train your body to respond more quickly by increasing the pace of exercise sooner in each progressive workout. Don't start at full throttle, but over time, train your body to respond to the exercise load more quickly. Your body adapts to the increasing quickness of the demands of your exercise by improving the quickness of your response.

Why do this? This is the natural state of exercise. Whether predator or prey, in the wild creatures must be able to accelerate to 100 percent capacity in a single heartbeat. Humans have lost this ability to accelerate, somewhat recently. More to the point, this is also the very best way to be prepared for and avoid disaster from the sudden increases in cardiac demand that cause heart attacks.

Intensity

Intensity simply refers to how hard you exercise. Intensity is what you should be monitoring and changing as you become fit. Remember, for any exercise program to continue to work over time, you must change something. If you perform the same exercise in the same way for more than a couple of weeks, your body has already adapted to the increased demands. You will cease to make any progress unless you challenge yourself further.

In the belief that they are building a stronger heart, many people increase the duration of exercise as they become more capable of exercising longer. But think about it! Your heart already has the ultimate endurance challenge — it must beat all the time, even when you're sleeping. Instead of working longer, strive to make your heart learn to pump more blood faster and harder for a short period of time.

You can use this principle safely as long as you increase the intensity in a controlled and gradual way. As your cardiac capacity increases, you can do more work without feeling any additional strain. If you walk or jog on a treadmill, about once a week you should pick up the pace a little or increase the slope by a little. If you're pedaling a bicycle, you need to pedal a little faster or add a little resistance.

Duration

You can also increase the challenge of your working by changing the duration of your exercise, but in the opposite direction of most exercisers. As your level of fitness improves, you need to decrease the duration of your workout. In other words, you cover the same distance in shorter and shorter times. You will find that by gradually shortening your intervals, it gets easier to increase the intensity with each session, and increasing intensity will continue to increase your capacity.

During your rest periods, don't stop entirely but keep moving at a gentle pace as you recover. Light activity keeps your blood circulating to replenish your muscles' depleted energy stores and removes accumulated lactic acid wastes. Studies show that your muscles recover faster with light activity than with complete immobility. For instance, if you sprint during your interval, you will keep moving at a walk or gentle trot for your rest period. You have a natural inclination to do this. If you listen to your body, you will want to keep moving after a sprint to "walk it off."

As you begin your PACE™ Program, work out just 10 to 20 minutes every other day. If you are getting in 20 minutes of exercise, you will want to divide your 20-minute workout into two 10-minute intervals. As you get into better shape, cut your exercise sessions down to 9 minutes; rest for three minutes, then workout another 9 minutes. Next, progress to three six-minute intervals with two minutes of rest in between each interval. Again, the principle is to cut the exercise length gradually as you gradually pick up the challenge. To get a feel for how progressively increasing the intensity as you decrease the duration plays out through time, take a look at the table, 8 Week Plan At-A-Glance on page 123.

Use Your Heart Rate to Measure Intensity

You can use your pulse rate, or the number of heartbeats per minute, as your heart's speedometer. It tells you how fast you're going, and whether you need to speed up or slow down to exercise in your optimal conditioning zone.

Target Pulse Ranges

Age	Max Heart Rate	Target Range
25	195	137-166
30	190	133-162
35	185	130-157
40	180	126-153
45	175	122-149
50	170	119-145
55	165	115-140
60	160	112-136
65	155	109-132
70	150	105-128
75	145	102-123
80	140	98-119
85	135	95-115
90	130	91-110

You can effectively challenge your heart by coaching it to beat at a pace that is 70 to 85 percent of its maximum safe rate. Your maximum heart rate is roughly equal to 220 minus your age.

Measure your heart rate any place on your body where you can feel your pulse. Two easy pulse points are the inside wrist and the carotid artery in the neck. Using a stopwatch, count your pulse for ten seconds, then multiply that number by six to get the number of beats per minute. Let's say you counted a pulse of 15 in 10 seconds. Multiply 15 times 6, and you'll calculate a heart rate of 90 beats per minute. You can also wear an exercise heart monitor that does the math for you, available over the Internet and from most fitness shops. You can even find wrist watch heart rate monitors at the big discount department store chains.

During exercise, if your pulse is less than your target range, speed up or work harder. If your pulse is more than your target range, slow down. For example, let's suppose you're a thirty-five year old running on the treadmill and your heart is beating 120 beats a minute. To get your heart beating within the target range of 130-157, you pick up the pace or increase the resistance. Suppose later during the workout, your pulse rate is 180. To get your heart beating within the target range of 130-157, you slow your pace or decrease the resistance.

EXERCISE CAUTION

Check with your doctor before starting an exercise program if any of the following apply to you:

- You haven't had a medical checkup in more than two years.
- You're over 50.
- You're more than 25 pounds overweight.
- You have high blood pressure.
- You've had a heart attack, rapid heart palpitations, or chest pain after exercise.
- You're taking heart medication.

- Your doctor told you that you have angina, fibrillation, tachycardia, an abnormal EKG, a heart murmur, rheumatic heart disease, or other heart problems.
- You have a blood relative who died of a heart attack before age sixty.
- You have asthma, emphysema, or any other lung condition.

Find Your PACE™

Build your exercise program around any activity that gives your heart and lungs a workout. Swimming, biking, stair-stepping, sprinting and elliptical machines are all good exercises for the heart and lungs. What form of exercise you chose will depend on your preferences and your level of fitness. You might want to alternate the various types of exercise to keep your routine fun and lower the chances of overuse injuries. You are most likely to stick with your program when you choose exercises you enjoy.

Here is a week-by-week outline of the PACE™ plan:

Weeks 1 and 2

Begin by developing an exercise routine based on activities you enjoy. Your goal is to perform this exercise for 20 minutes at a time at low intensity. If you can't exercise for 20 minutes without stopping, rest as needed. As you're starting out write down what you do. It is helpful to determine your current level of fitness to use as a baseline to track your progress.

In the second week, begin experimenting with the pace. Push yourself a little harder and then ease up a bit. Vary your pace as much as you feel comfortable.

As you play with the pace, begin to develop an internal scale of how intensely you exercise. Use a scale of 1 to 10, where 1 or 2 is a leisurely pace, all the way up to full throttle at 9 or 10.

Week 1
- Exercise for 20 minutes at a comfortable intensity level of 2 or 3.

Week 2
- Exercise for 20 minutes at varying intensity levels recording your pace and how hard it feels.

Weeks 3 and 4

In weeks 3 and 4, increase the amount of work you do in the same amount of time. If you exercise on a treadmill or cycling machine, push yourself to cover more distance in the same time. Your workout now consists of two intervals, with a rest period in between. During the periods of rest, you don't have to be completely inactive. You will do better to keep moving at low intensity while you recover.

Week 3
- Exercise for 9 minutes at intensity level 3
- Rest for 2 minutes
- Exercise for 9 minutes of exercise at intensity level 4

Week 4
- Exercise for 8 minutes at intensity level 4
- Rest for 4 minutes
- Exercise for 8 minutes of exercise at intensity level 5

Weeks 5 and 6

In weeks 5 and 6, exercise more intensely during three somewhat shorter intervals.

Week 5
- Exercise for 6 minutes of exercise at intensity level 3
- Rest for 2 minutes
- Exercise for 6 minutes at intensity level 5

- Rest for 2 minutes
- Exercise for 6 minutes at intensity level 4

Week 6

Decrease each exercise period to 5 minutes, while you increase the intensity by one level. Since you are working a little harder, allow yourself 3 minutes of leisurely-paced rest to recover between intervals.

Weeks 7 and 8

t's time to put the accelerating component of your PACE™ program into play. Your goal is to take less and less time to reach the point of your greatest effort. The result is that you complete more intervals during the same time and you increase the level quicker. The shorter your intervals of greatest intensity, the faster you condition your body for maximal capacity.

Week 7
- Exercise for 4 minutes at intensity level 4
- Rest for 2 minutes
- Exercise for 3 minutes at intensity level 6
- Rest for 2 minutes
- Exercise for 2 minutes at intensity level 7
- Rest for 3 minutes
- Exercise for 3 minutes at intensity level 5

Week 8

Now you will shorten your first interval a little and increase the intensity of your second interval a bit. You are "accelerating" your challenge with your highest effort occurring earlier.
- Exercise for 3 minutes at intensity level 4
- Rest for 2 minutes
- Exercise for 3 minutes at intensity level 7
- Rest for 2 minutes
- Exercise for 3 minutes at intensity level 7
- Rest for 2 minutes
- Exercise for 3 minutes at intensity level 5

Progressively Accelerating Cardiopulmonary Exertion™ PACE™: 8-Week Plan At-A-Glance

Activity	Week 1	Week 2	Week 3	Week 4
Exercise	Exercise 20 min	Exercise 20 min	Exercise 9 min	Exercise 8 min
Intensity Level	Level 3 or 4	Varying	Level 3	Level 4
Rest			2 min	4 min
Exercise			Exercise 9 min	Exercise 8 min
Intensity Level			Level 4	Level 5
Activity	**Week 5**	**Week 6**	**Week 7**	**Week 8**
Exercise	Exercise 6 min	Exercise 5 min	Exercise 4 min	Exercise 3 min
Intensity Level	Level 3	Level 4	Level 4	Level 4
Rest	Rest 2 min	Rest 2 min	Rest 2 min	Rest 2 min
Exercise	Exercise 6 min	Exercise 5 min	Exercise 3 min	Exercise 3 min
Intensity Level	Level 5	Level 6	Level 6	Level 7
Rest	Rest 2 min	Rest 3 min	Rest 2 min	Rest 2 min
Exercise	Exercise 6 min	Exercise 5 min	Exercise 2 min	Exercise 3 min
Intensity Level	Level 4	Level 5	Level 7	Level 7
Rest			Rest 3 min	Rest 2 min
Exercise			Exercise 3 min	Exercise 3 min
Intensity Level			Level 5	Level 5

Implement the Full Tilt Program

As you continue to pick up the PACE™, increase the intensity of your workout and the number of exercise intervals. At the same time, shorten the length of your exercise sessions. You may be doing three five-minute intervals with two three-minutes rests. As you progress, shorten the length of your exercise intervals to four, three, two, then one minute. Work a little harder during these shorter exercise sessions. When you get used to PACE™ and use it to your full advantage, your workout sessions usually last less than 14 minutes!

Here is a sample workout plan to advance your PACE™ when you have conditioned yourself to the challenge. It takes only 10 minutes:

Interval Training

Interval 1
• Exercise for 1 minute at intensity level 5
• Rest 1 minute at intensity level 3
Interval 2
• Exercise for 1 minute at intensity level 6
• Rest for 1 minute at intensity level 4
Interval 3
• Exercise for 45 seconds at intensity level 7
• Rest 1 minute at intensity level 4
Interval 4
• Exercise 45 seconds at intensity level 8
• Rest 1 minute at intensity level 3
Interval 5
• Exercise 30 seconds at intensity level 9
• Rest for 2 minutes at intensity level 2

When you become conditioned well enough to do it, exercising for just 30 seconds at an intensity level of 9 or 10 will seem like a surprisingly long time. In fact, your body cannot sustain exercise at this level much longer because your muscles need more oxygen than your body can supply. But this is exactly why it pays off! This rate of exercise is training your heart and blood vessels to deliver more oxygen faster.

DON'T MAKE IT DIFFICULT

The most common mistake beginners make is assuming that they must work at an uncomfortable level of exertion to get results. This is an understandable interpretation since you will be focusing your attention on your exercise intensity, but it is not necessary.

The point is to start with what is a comfortable level of exertion for you. As you improve your fitness, this same level of activity will become easier for you. Now you make use of your added capacity by increasing the level of the exercise. This will coach your body into increasing your exercise capacity further. With this week-by-week gradual progression of your workout as your body responds, you do not feel an uncomfortable or painful perceived level of exertion.

MEN AND CYCLING

There are studies that link long-distance cycling to impotency. The key phrase is long distance. Most of the research studied men who cycled for several hours every day. Fortunately, there is no evidence of any risk if you cycle for short duration.

When a man sits on a bicycle seat, his groin supports the entire weight of his body. This puts intense pressure in the area near the genitals, which contains the nerves and arteries that transmit feeling and blood to the genitals. Prolonged pressure can cause genital numbness and even temporary impotency.

You can build reserve capacity in your heart, lungs, and muscles in as little as ten minutes a day. There is no need to sit on a bicycle seat for an extended amount of time. Limit your cycling to less than three hours a week.

If you like cycling and are still concerned, vary your activities. Cycle a few times a week and do other forms of exercise you like during the rest of the week. Also, check with bicycle companies that recently marketed new seats designed specifically to take pressure off the genitals.

Strengthen Your Frame

Let's get something clear that often gets confused. Muscle size and strength are not the same things. Yes, of course, the two are related, but modern day bodybuilders create so much muscular hypertrophy that they can hardly get out of their own way.

In contrast, you may need to increase the size of your muscles. Muscle wasting has its consequences in aging. In that case, resistance training may be your best course. It is a scientific way to apply overload to isolated muscles. Since you can easily manipulate the resistance by incrementally increasing the weight, you can perpetuate the stimulus for muscle growth.

You can use your body composition measurements from Chapter 5, Measure Your Real Heart Health, to determine if you need to build or restore muscle mass. If your muscle mass is low, you will find a program for quick and efficient muscle building in Chapter 11, Individualize *Your Doctor's Heart Cure*.

But in years of practical application, one glaring limitation of weight training remains: You're not really training anything. It's more "untraining" your muscles; it teaches them to tense. This tends to create unnatural patterns of movement, sets you up for injuries, and is not the best way to build practical strength that you can use.

Exercises that put your body through "functional" natural patterns of movement train your entire circuit from thought to action. This neuromuscular education is essential if you want that new muscle to be capable of doing anything. Whenever you call on your muscles in real life, they move against the resistance of your own bodyweight. Before weight training became the rule, we called these bodyweight exercises calisthenics. They are still the best way to build functional strength.

Your prehistoric ancestors had to run, jump, climb, and fight in their daily pursuit of food and security. You can develop the extraordinary functional strength of wild animals by using your own bodyweight.

Bodybuilders can develop massive muscles through intensive resistance training, but gymnasts, acrobats, swimmers, sprinters, and athletes in many disciplines develop better functional muscle capacity. They have greater practical strength in response to the demands of their bodies in motion.

Remember, your cardiovascular system has muscle, too. These optimal exercises for growing your muscular strength will also help to strengthen the muscles of your heart, the muscles lining your blood vessels and the muscles expanding your lungs.

Common Sense Calisthenics

In daily life, your muscles work against the resistance of your body-weight. Despite the fancy exercise equipment in gyms, calisthenics remain the best way to build strength that you can use. Calisthenics are also much more effective in strengthening ligaments and tendons.[1] To build strength that you can use work against your own body's weight.

Strengthen Your Foundation: Exercise Your Legs & Lower Body

Let's start from the bottom up. Your lower body is more important for functional strength than your upper body. For both men and women, there appears to be little benefit to creating oversized muscles in the arms, chest and shoulders, and having a muscular imbalance between the upper and lower body can harm joints (especially shoulders and neck) and posture later in life.[2]

Your biggest muscles are your quadriceps on the front of your thighs, followed by your hamstrings on the back of your thighs and the gluteus muscles in your buttocks, meaning your three biggest muscles all work to flex and extend your hip. If you want to maximize your exercise's effect on your total body strength, go to the muscles that nature designed to be the strongest and work them first.

- **Do alternating lunges:** Stand straight with your hands on your hips and your feet together. Take a long step forward with your left leg and bend your right knee down to the ground. Straighten up as you now step forward with your right foot, returning to a standing position with your feet together. Repeat and alternate legs as you "walk" down a hallway or across a room.

- **Squat:** With your feet shoulder-width apart and pointing slightly away from each other, move your buttocks down and backward as if you were about to sit on a low stool. Keep moving downward until your thighs are parallel to the floor. Although you want to keep your back straight for good posture, there is no need to keep your back upright, perpendicular to the floor. It is natural and necessary for good balance and more comfortable if you allow yourself to bend at the waist leaning your upper body forward as you push your buttocks back and down. Keep your heels flat on the floor.

- **Take squat leaps:** Stand straight with your hands on your hips and your feet shoulder-width apart. Squat down until your legs are almost at right angles. Now jump straight up as high as you can like a rocket launching.

Strengthen Your Core: Exercise Your Abdomen & Lower Back

Now let's concentrate on your abdomen. Strong abdominal muscles help prevent pain and injury in the lower back. Remember, these exercises alone won't eliminate that spare tire. You'll need to improve your diet to go along with your new exercise program. Building powerful core muscle groups supports functional strength. These muscles improve your breath, posture, and the mechanics of motion.

- **Crunch your midsection:** Lie on your back. Place your palms on the floor and move your hands underneath your buttocks and press the small of your back firmly on the floor. Slowly raise your head and feet slightly off the ground. Hold for one second and slowly lower them. Repeat. You can vary the muscles you use by lifting your legs higher, by crossing one leg over the other at the knee, or by raising only your head.

- **Leg Levers:** Lying on your back, start with your legs six inches above the ground, lift your legs about another foot higher and bring them back down to the starting position. Repeat.

- **Back Flutter Kicks:** Lie on your back and alternate raising each leg to about two or three feet off the ground. Repeat.

- **Scissors:** Lie on your back and raise your legs a few inches off the ground. Now spread your legs apart and bring them back together. Repeat. Your legs look like scissors opening and closing.

Strengthen Your Upper Body

Use your own bodyweight to challenge your upper body as well. Engaging in full-range of motion activities will build your practical strength. Your muscles will become useful to you and power your ability to do everyday activities like lifting a heavy package or moving a couch.

When you work your upper body, focus on your back more than your chest and arms. This does more to prevent injury than spending time on your extremities.

- **Pushups:** Pushups work your entire upper body, strengthening the pectorals of the chest, the deltoids of the shoulders, the triceps of the arms, and the muscles of the upper, middle, and lower back. Lie face down on the ground. Place your hands a bit wider than shoulder-width apart. Place your feet together, and straighten your back. Lower yourself until you're almost touching the ground. If you have trouble at first, try doing them with your knees on the ground and your feet in the air. When you master the traditional version, play with clapping your hands between each pushup.

- **Arm Haulers:** Lie on your stomach and stretch your arms in front of you. Raise your arms and legs off the floor. Then sweep your arms all the way back to your thighs, as if you're doing the breaststroke. Finish by returning your arms back to the starting position.

- **Pull-ups:** With the traditional pull-ups, you raise and lower your weight on a bar. You can vary the width of your grip on the bar; a wide grip widens your back for more of a V-taper muscle formation.

Have your palms facing out for a traditional pull-up to strengthen the muscles of the middle back. If you grip the bar with your palms facing you, you are doing a chin-up. Chin-ups also use the back, but they recruit your biceps as well.

- **Dips:** You can do these between two chairs or two desks, or a set of parallel bars. While putting one hand on each object, lift your feet off the ground, then slowly lower yourself until your elbows are at a 90-degree angle. Pause then slowly raise yourself. This exercise is great for the chest, middle back, and triceps.

DESIGN A WORKOUT PLAN

You can combine these exercises in many different ways. For example, you can split up your exercise by major muscle groups, work a different muscle group each day and do three sets of 10 repetitions for each exercise you choose for the day.

You can find more on the Internet or at the library. Decide on some favorites and then create your program. Also remember to include your PACE™ program in your regimen.

A Favorite Workout Plan

Day 1	PACE™
Day 2	Legs and Abs
Day 3	PACE™
Day 4	Rest
Day 5	PACE™
Day 6	Back, Chest and Arms
Day 7	PACE™

Plan to Succeed

It is helpful to keep a log of your health plan. There is no better pre-dictor of who will succeed at reaching their goals than whether or not they are willing to keep a log. If you want to reach your fitness goals, write down what you plan to do – then write down what you actually do. A written record of your workouts helps you measure your progress.

YOUR ACTION PLAN

- Exercise your heart, lung and blood vessel capacity by following the PACE™ program.
- Build functional strength with bodyweight exercises.

Footnotes Chapter 7

1 LaStayo P, Ewy GA, Pierotti DD, et al. The positive effects of negative work: increased muscle strength and decreased fall risk in a frail elderly population. *Journal of Gerontology and Biological Science and Medical Science.* 2003 May; 58(5):M419-424.

2 Brose A, Parise G and Ternoppoisy, MA. Creatine supplementation enhances isometric strength and body composition improvements following strength exer-cise training in older adults. *Journal of Gerontology and Biological Science and Medical Science.* 2003 Jan; 58(1):11-19.

8

Energize Your Heart:
The Miracle of CoQ10

The human body requires adequate levels of coenzyme Q10 (CoQ10) to survive. It's no secret that this essential antioxidant is important to maintain a healthy heart. But there is one dirty little secret about CoQ10 that drug manufacturers don't want you to know: Cholesterol-lowering statin drugs slash the levels of CoQ10 in the body.

While these drugs reduce the production of cholesterol in the liver, they also lower the production of CoQ10. In fact, studies found that statin drugs lower CoQ10 levels by as much as 40 percent.[1]

Drug companies know about this dangerous side effect. One company even developed a statin-CoQ10 combination drug to offset the CoQ10 stripped from the body but have decided to hold the patent without releasing the nutrient drug combination to the public. Clearly the companies recognize that their drugs drain the body of CoQ10, and they have done nothing to educate physicians and patients about this very real danger of taking statins. Instead, they downplay this fact in hopes that the news about this side effect does not interfere with drug sales.

Unfortunately, most doctors don't know enough about the link between statin drugs and CoQ10 to recommend that their patients take supplements. Some misinformed doctors even discourage the use of CoQ10 and other nutritional supplements altogether.

Recently, a retired chorus line dancer from New York City came to the Center for Health and Wellness for the first time with high blood pressure even though she was taking two blood pressure medications and a statin drug. She said she felt constant fatigue and increasing trouble remembering. When her blood level of CoQ10 was measured, it was lower than 95% of the population. After taking 200 mg of CoQ10 supplement daily for a couple of months, she was able to stop both blood pressure medications and now maintains a normal blood pressure. She also reported feeling "energized" and she recovered her memory.

She returned to the cardiologist to tell him the good news. She showed him the remarkable nutrient that normalized her blood pressure better than the drugs. Rather than rejoice in her success, he became irate, told her the CoQ10 could not possibly help her blood pressure and threw her CoQ10 in the trash. Incredibly, this is not the only story like this one. Together they reveal a troubling double standard. Most doctors are well informed of the uses and benefits of drugs but uninformed and suspicious of nutritional solutions. Yet more than 100 studies show the cardiac benefits of CoQ10.

In this chapter, you'll find out how and why CoQ10 works to strengthen the heart. Since it is difficult to get optimal levels of this substance from the typical modern American diet, you'll also discover how to use CoQ10 supplements in your heart-healthy routine.

Discover the Remarkable Benefits of CoQ10

At the Center for Health and Wellness, *more than half the patients who were taking drugs for high blood pressure were able to stop their medication once they began taking CoQ10.* CoQ10 is nothing short of a miracle heart energizer.

CoQ10 is an essential cofactor your body uses to derive energy. You cannot survive without it. CoQ10 is a powerful anti-oxidant present in every cell in your body. Because of its ubiquitous presence (it's everywhere!), you may see it referred to as ubiquinone.

CoQ10 is essential for the normal function of all your major organs. It is especially important to the energy-guzzling organs, like your heart, brain, kidneys, and liver. CoQ10 provides your body with "high octane" fuel. Also, this co-enzyme gives the body five more vital benefits! CoQ10:

1. Destroys free radicals before they can damage your cell membranes.

2. Prevents arteriosclerosis by reducing the accumulation of oxidized fat

in your blood vessels.

3. Eases heart disease, high blood pressure, and high cholesterol.
4. Reduces chest pain and improves exercise tolerance in patients with chronic stable angina.
5. Regulates the rhythm of the heart rate.

Pump Up Your Mitochondria

CoQ10 works like magic on mitochondria. Mitochondria are the structures in your cells that manufacture energy at the cellular level. Virtually every cell in the body has its own energy-producing mitochondria designed to meet the needs of each individual cell. (There are no mitochondria in red blood cells or the lens of the eye.) Most cells contain between 500 and 2,000 mitochondria; the highest concentrations of mitochondria exist in the busiest cells of the body, including the brain, heart, kidneys, and additional hardworking organs.

Energy production at the cellular level begins when the body turns the food we eat into nutrients (glucose, amino acids, and fatty acids) the mitochondria can use to produce energy. Within the cells, the mitochondria – through a multi-step process scientists refer to as the Krebs cycle – manufacture adenosine triphosphate (ATP). ATP is literally the body's source of energy. ATP is the fuel cells burn to perform their tasks.

To make energy, the mitochondria use plenty of CoQ10, which helps in the chemical reactions required for energy production. This is essential to keep the powerhouses of the cells – the mitochondria – working efficiently. In effect, the CoQ10 provides a virtual Fountain of Youth for the cells.

When cells run out of CoQ10, the mitochondria simply cannot produce enough energy to meet the body's demands. When the body is well stocked with CoQ10, it can operate efficiently. When stockpiles of CoQ10 run low, the mitochondria are less efficient and they may produce adenosine diphosphate (ADP), which is a less potent fuel. Over time, running your body on cheap fuel will take its toll, damaging the mitochondria and contributing to a growing sense of fatigue.

When our bodies are young, our mitochondria work tirelessly to produce the abundant energy associated with youth. Over the years, however, our mitochondria age and show signs of wear and tear, just as the rest of the body does. The mitochondria can grow hard and less efficient at producing ATP. When the mitochondria break down, they produce less energy. If this happens long enough, you experience chronic fatigue. This makes the heart weak and inefficient. This systemic energy crisis can compromise the immune system as a whole, leaving our bodies more vulnerable to attack from bacteria, viruses, and additional pathogens.

A number of studies found that people who suffer from ailments associated with aging – including cardiovascular disease, Parkinson's disease, and Alzheimer's disease – all tend to have abnormally low levels of CoQ10 and high levels of mitochondria failure. The Center for Health and Wellness has measured hundreds of patients' CoQ10 levels, with some surprising results.

- Young people (those in their twenties and younger) almost always have adequate levels of CoQ10.
- CoQ10 deficiencies are common in people in their forties and beyond.
- Long-duration endurance exercisers tend to have lower levels of CoQ10.
- Deficiencies in CoQ10 are very common in patients with heart disease, high blood pressure, diabetes or low HDL cholesterols.
- CoQ10 levels are often low in those avoiding red meat and extremely low in strict vegans.

If you are in one of these categories, as hundreds of patients discovered, CoQ10 supplements can make a dramatic difference in your energy level and cardiovascular health.

Discovery of CoQ10

Dr. Frederick Crane, the so-called Father of CoQ10 research, discovered CoQ10 at the University of Wisconsin in 1953. Crane initially assumed that the substance was related to the A vitamins, but later realized it was something altogether different. He continued to conduct research on the substance and in 1957 found it in the mitochondria of cow heart muscle.

In 1958, biochemist Karl Folkers, Ph.D., director of the Institute for Biomedical Research at the University of Texas at Austin, and researchers at a pharmaceutical company identified the chemical structure of CoQ10, and soon developed a way to synthesize it. At the time, scientists did not appreciate the significance of their discovery. Since CoQ10 was a natural substance, it could not be patented, and it was expensive to produce. The pharmaceutical company sold the technology for the production of CoQ10 to Japanese researchers.

During the late 1950s and 1960s, Japanese researchers experimented with CoQ10 and its role in the body. They soon discovered that CoQ10 was effective in the treatment of congestive heart failure, a condition that does not respond well to traditional treatments. Western researchers paid little attention to this CoQ10 breakthrough. They believed the answer to heart disease was open heart surgery and other surgical solutions, rather than a simple nutritional supplement.

Researchers also found that CoQ10 is a powerful anti-oxidant. Anti-oxidants help the body neutralize free radicals in the cell. Free radical damage contributes to a range of diseases and medical problems, including heart disease, cancer, Alzheimer's disease, arthritis, and more problems associated with aging. Free radicals are one of the metabolic byproducts of energy production in the cells. CoQ10 appears to protect the cells and the mitochondria by cleaning up these free radicals before they can damage the cells. Now, even Western researchers appreciate the importance of CoQ10 in both energy production and the health of the cells.

Research of CoQ10

Studies find that CoQ10 protects and strengthens the heart, protects the brain, and revitalizes the immune system. There are more than 100 studies at major universities and hospitals linking CoQ10 deficiency with heart disease. Additional studies show taking CoQ10 revitalizes heart function and can dramatically relieve heart disease symptoms. Consider the evidence.

Heal Your Heart with CoQ10

Some of the most impressive studies on CoQ10 researched the role of the supplement in the treatment of cardiovascular disease. In a landmark study, Dr. Folkers and his colleagues found CoQ10 deficiency in a majority of people with heart disease. Researchers measured the levels of CoQ10 in heart tissue biopsies. And they found low levels of CoQ10 in 50 to 75 percent of patients with various types of heart disease.[2]

The next round of studies looked at whether taking supplemental CoQ10 could help prevent or reverse heart disease. Since the 1970s, more than 50 studies demonstrated the effectiveness of CoQ10 in the treatment of people with heart disease. Dr. Folkers and Dr. Peter Langsjoen, a cardiologist in Tyler, Texas, conducted a remarkable study between 1985 and 1993. They observed 424 people who received CoQ10 and conventional medicine treatments for heart disease. Doctors then assessed patient progress according to the New York Heart Association functional scale. The heart disease ratings range from I (the least serious) to IV (the most serious). After taking CoQ10, 58 percent of the patients improved one category, 28 percent moved up two categories, and 1.2 percent moved up three categories! In addition, 43 percent of the patients cut back or eliminated their cardiac medication.

CoQ10 also helps lower blood pressure. A double-blind, placebo-controlled study in the *Journal of Human Hypertension* followed two groups of people with hypertension. One group took CoQ10 for eight weeks while the other group took a placebo. The COQ10 group showed a significant reduction in blood pressure.[3] *Molecular Aspects of Medicine* reported another fascinating study about patients taking CoQ10 and prescription drugs for high blood pressure. Researchers found that more than half of all patients on blood pressure drugs were able to stop using their medications when they began taking supplemental CoQ10. In a University of Texas study, people with high blood pressure took oral CoQ10. Within one month, they experienced marked improvements in blood pressure. Overall, 51 percent of subjects were able to discontinue their blood pressure medication.[4]

CoQ10 offers results with very little risk of unwanted side effects.

Many medications for cardiovascular disease have unpleasant side effects, including fatigue, nausea, and dizziness. CoQ10 offers many of the same health benefits as prescription drugs do – without their harmful side effects.

Reverse Congestive Heart Failure

The best treatment for congestive heart failure is a daily dose of CoQ10. It works better than any other medication prescribed. Many cases of cardiovascular disease completely resolve when patients begin taking CoQ10.

Deprive your heart of CoQ10 and its available energy declines, leading to a decrease in the volume of blood your heart can pump. If your heart pumps less blood than it receives, fluid backs up and your heart swells like a water balloon. We call this congestive heart failure.

Congestive heart failure can affect either the right or left side of the heart. The left side pumps oxygen-rich blood from the lungs to the rest of the body. The right side of the heart pumps the oxygen-depleted blood from the body back to the lungs that replenish the oxygen. When the left side of the heart is damaged, the blood backs up into the lungs, causing wheezing and shortness of breath (even during rest), fatigue, sleep disturbances, and a dry, hacking, non-productive cough when lying down. When the right side of the heart is damaged, the blood collects in the legs and liver, causing swollen feet and ankles, swollen neck veins, pain below the ribs, fatigue, and lethargy. People with congestive heart failure tend to have abnormally low levels of CoQ10. They also have many problems or abnormalities with the mitochondria of their cells, probably caused by the low levels of healing CoQ10.

CoQ10 is important in the treatment of congestive heart failure, a disease that is often fatal. While some traditional medications can improve heart function temporarily, they often delay death by no more than a few month or years at best. The five-year survival rate for people with congestive heart failure is 50 percent, and many people with the condition suffer from severe functional disabilities.

CoQ10 offers hope for people with congestive heart failure. CoQ10 changes how the heart functions and strengthens cells. Patients with congestive heart failure can dramatically prolong their lives by taking CoQ10. In one study, taking CoQ10 cut the average yearly death rate of patients with heart failure by 26 to 59 percent.[5] Many patients reverse their heart failure by taking regular doses of CoQ10.

Ease Angina Pectoris

About 3 million Americans suffer from angina, a painful attack that occurs when the heart muscle does not get enough oxygen. (The medical term for this is myocardial ischemia.) Physical exertion, emotional upset, excessive excitement, or even digestion of a heavy meal can trigger angina attacks in people whose hearts are damaged by high blood pressure and coronary artery disease. Angina attacks often serve as painful reminders that the heart is damaged, and a full-blown heart attack may follow unless steps are taken to mend your ailing heart. The good news is you can mend it.

CoQ10 helps people with angina pectoris. As part of a double-blind study (one in which neither the doctor nor the patients know who gets the medication and who gets the placebo), 12 people with angina pectoris took 150 mg CoQ10 daily for four weeks. Patients taking CoQ10 experienced a 53 percent reduction in the frequency of their angina attacks, compared to patients who took the placebo. In addition, those people taking CoQ10 could exercise on a treadmill a lot longer than they could before they started taking CoQ10.[6]

Recover from Heart Surgery

CoQ10 produces impressive results during recovery from heart surgery. A series of fascinating Australian studies demonstrate that CoQ10 may create youthful performance in older hearts.[7] In the first study, researchers placed hearts taken from old and young rats in a device to keep them beating artificially. The researchers then raced the hearts under excessive stress. The extreme stress accelerated the heart rate to more than 500 beats per minute for two hours. At the end of the test, the young hearts recovered 45 percent of their initial function, while the old hearts recovered only 17 percent of their function.

During the second phase, one group of rats received CoQ10 for six weeks, while the other group had a placebo. Researchers then sacrificed the rats and duplicated the heartbeat marathon. The young rat hearts performed the same, whether they had received CoQ10 earlier or not. The old hearts that had received the CoQ10, on the other hand, recovered at the same rate as the young hearts. In other words, the hearts of old rats that received CoQ10 performed just as well as the hearts of young rats.

How does this discovery apply to human hearts? We know that elders do not generally tolerate heart surgery well. That option is often closed to people over 70. We believe the problem stems from "reperfusion injury". This injury occurs because during open heart surgery, the surgical team must stop the heart to operate on it, then re-starts the heart when they've finished. The heart-lung machine continues to circulate blood to the body during the operation. During the surgery, the heart lacks oxygen and blood, just as it does during a heart attack. When the circulation is re-started, the body experiences a rush of oxygen that causes extreme free radical damage to heart tissue. Free radicals are unstable cells that tend to "steal" electrons from neighboring cells. We know that CoQ10 helps neutralize these free radicals. Could it prevent damage to the heart caused by stopping and starting the heart during open heart surgery?

To test the theory, cardiologists bathed heart tissue in a solution that provided it with oxygen and glucose. Next, they ran an electric current through the solution to cause the heart tissue to "beat." Researchers then measured the strength of the heart muscle contractions.

They then deprived the heart tissue of oxygen and glucose for an hour to simulate the experience of open heart surgery. Then they restored the oxygen and glucose, causing the release of free radicals. In this situation, the younger heart muscles recovered 70 percent of their strength while the older heart muscles regained just 49 percent of their strength.

To test the impact of CoQ10 on the heart, the researchers administered CoQ10 to the heart tissue for 30 minutes before repeating the oxygen- and glucose-deprivation experiment. As in the rat heart experiment, the old hearts showed marked improvement. In fact, old heart tissue pre-treated with CoQ10 actually recovered an astounding 72 percent of its contraction strength, slightly better than the recovery rate of the young hearts.[8]

In these experiments, CoQ10 helps old heart recover as well as young hearts do. But don't think that CoQ10 is effective only in older hearts. Research suggests it has other benefits to both young and old hearts alike. CoQ10 can help prevent free radicals from damaging the heart in the first place. Other studies have shown that CoQ10 can lower oxidation of cholesterol and incidence of heart attacks.

The combination of CoQ10 and carnitine offers more dramatic benefits. Together, CoQ10 and carnitine help the body maintain healthy levels of cholesterol and other body lipids. CoQ10 lowers overall cholesterol levels, while carnitine lowers triglyceride levels and raises HDL (the protective form of cholesterol).

Protect Your Brain with CoQ10

CoQ10 is in high concentrations in the brain where it helps generate much needed energy. Brain levels begin declining at the age of 20, and are lowest in stroke victims and those with neuro-degenerative diseases. There is growing evidence that CoQ10 is neuro-protective and may stave off the difficult problems of loss of memory with age.

Recent research focused on the effect of CoQ10 on degenerative neurological diseases, such as Huntington's disease and Lou Gehrig's disease (also known as amyotrophic lateral sclerosis, or ALS). For the most part, doctors can offer little hope to people suffering from these conditions, but CoQ10 may hold some promise for healing.

Research at Massachusetts General Hospital in Boston looked at the role of CoQ10 in preventing neurological disorders. First, researchers administered a brain poison to older animals, to bring on a physical state similar to that caused by Huntington's disease or ALS in humans. Animals that took supplemental CoQ10 experienced much less damage caused by the poison, compared with the animals that did not receive the CoQ10. Clinical trials on humans are under way to examine whether CoQ10 can help prevent or stall the course of these illnesses in people.

Strengthen Your Immune System with CoQ10

A number of studies show that CoQ10 helps strengthen the immune response, especially in people whose immune systems are weak. How does CoQ10 work its magic on immunity? Research suggests that CoQ10's antioxidant power may directly protect the immune cells from free radical damage. CoQ10 may regulate the genes that control cell activity. CoQ10 may help facilitate communication among the immune-system cells. This allows them to offer a timely and powerful response to any potential threat.

CoQ10 may help fight cancer by strengthening the immune system. In 2000, researchers found that people suffering from cancer had lower levels of CoQ10 in the blood than people without cancer did.[9] Additional research found CoQ10 makes immune cells – known as T-cells – more efficient. T-cells seek and destroy cancer cells in the body.[10]

Get Plenty of CoQ10

Your body has several ways to obtain CoQ10 to meet your physical demands. Only very young and vigorously healthy people seem to make enough internally. As we age, we rapidly become more dependent on dietary sources. Your gut can absorb it from the foods you eat, but it has become difficult to get optimal levels of CoQ10 from the typical modern diet.

Organ meats of animals are the primary food sources of CoQ10. Can you remember the last time you dined on deer kidney, goat brains, or lamb heart? Even if you did, the organs of wild, grass-fed animals have up to ten times more CoQ10 than the organs of grain-fed animals. Unless you regularly consume wild game or eat internal organs of grass-fed animals, it is difficult to maintain good blood levels of CoQ10 from dietary sources alone. This modern predicament is the strongest case for supplementation. Here is a simple guide to dosing to be reasonably sure your body is getting adequate CoQ10 to produce energy for your organs and to protect your heart from common deficiencies.

- If you are over 30, take 30 milligrams of CoQ10 per day.
- If you are over 60, increase the dose to 60 milligrams.
- If you have high blood pressure, heart disease, gingivitis, memory loss, chronic fatigue, or are a vegetarian, increase your dose to 100 milligrams a day.
- If you take cholesterol-lowering "statin" drugs, such as Mevacor, Zocor, and Lipitor, take at least 100 milligrams of CoQ10 a day. Remember: prescription drugs block the body's production of CoQ10.

You can buy CoQ10 in the form of tablets, chewable wafers, or gel caps. Powdered capsules are not as well absorbed. Gel caps or chewable forms are absorbed better. When you squeeze a gel cap you can feel liquid inside. Because CoQ10 is a fat-soluble nutrient, take it with fat for optimal absorption.

You can take it when you eat dairy, eggs, fish or meat. You can even take it with a teaspoon of olive oil or fish oil. Grass-fed red meat, eggs and cod liver oil make the best fat choices to take with your CoQ10 because they contain CoQ10 naturally.

CoQ10 has no toxicity even at high doses in animals or humans. Any ill effects are minor and rare, usually nothing more than mild nausea. This can occur in groups of people taking any pill, even an empty gelatin capsule. You minimize this effect by taking CoQ10 with meals when you have food in your stomach.

If you take CoQ10, let your doctor know and monitor the favorable health benefits such as reduction in abnormally high blood pressures. If you take cardiovascular prescription drugs, ask your doctor whether you can reduce your dependence on these medications. To avoid the dangerous effects of abruptly discontinuing certain medications, change your medication only under the supervision of your physician.

CoQ10 Can Help Parkinson's Disease

A new study in *Archives of Neurology* shows that taking CoQ10 supplements helps patients with Parkinson's disease maintain mental function. In the 80-patient, 16-month study, those taking the highest doses of CoQ10 had the least loss of mental function. Those taking 1,200 mg had a 44% less decline in normal daily functions. (Shuts, Arch Neurol, 2002)

People with Parkinson's disease often have very low levels of CoQ10. Further testing is necessary to know if CoQ10 supplementation reduces the risk of developing Parkinson's disease.

ACTION PLAN

 Take 30 milligrams of CoQ10 daily if you're in good health.

 Take 100 milligrams of CoQ10 daily if you have heart disease.

 Take your CoQ10 supplement with food or a teaspoon of almond butter, olive oil or fish oil to maximize absorption.

Footnotes Chapter 8

1 Ghirlanda G, Oradei A, Manto A, et al. Evidence of plasma CoQ10-lowering effect of HMG-COA reductase inhibitors: a double-blind, placebo-controlled study. *Journal of Clinical Pharmacology.* 1993 Mar; 33(3):226-229.

2 Folkers K, Wolaniuk J, Simonsen R, et al. Biochemical rationale and the cardiac response of patients with muscle disease to therapy with coenzyme Q10. *Proceedings of the National Academy of Science.* 1985 Jul; 82(13):4513-4516.

3 Singh RB, Niaz MA, Rostogi SS, et al. Effect of hydrosoluble coenzyme Q10 on blood pressure in hypertensive patients with coronary artery disease. *Journal of Human Hypertension.* 1999 Mar; 13(3):203-208.

4 Langsjoen P, Langsjoen P, Willis R and Folkers K. Treatment of essential hypertension with coenzyme Q10. *Molecular Aspects of Medicine.* 1994; 15 Suppl:S265-272.

5 Langsjoen P.H. et al. Long-term efficacy and safety of coenzyme Q10 therapy for idiopathic dilated cardiomyopathy. *American Journal of Cardiology.* 1990; 65:521-523.

6 Kamikawa T, Kobayashi A, Yamashita T, et al. Effects of coenzyme Q10 on exercise tolerance in chronic stable angina pectoris. *American Journal of Cardiology.* 1995 Aug 1; 56(4):247-251.

7 Rosenfeldt FL, Pepe S, Linnane A, et al. Coenzyme Q10 protects the aging heart against stress: Studies in rats, human tissues, and patients. *Annals of New York Academy of Science.* 2002 Apr; 959:355-359.

8 Jeejeebhoy F, Keith M, Freeman M, et al. Nutritional supplementation with MyoVive repletes essential cardiac myocyte nutrients and reduces left ventricular size in patients with left ventricular dysfunction. *American Heart Journal.* 2002 Jun; 143(6):1092-1100.

9 Portakal O, Ozkaya O, Erden Inal M, et al. Coenzyme concentrations and antioxidant status in tissues of breast cancer patients. *Clinical Biochemistry.* 2000 Jun; 33(4):279-284.

10 Folkers K, Morita M and McRee J Jr. The activities of coenzyme Q10 and vitamin B6 for immune responses. *Biochemical and Biophysical Research Communications.* 1993 May 28; 193(1):88-92.

9

Give Your Heart the Four Nutrients It Needs

In medical school, physicians receive very little training in nutrition. Traditional medical education focuses on disease rather than health. As a result, most doctors remain woefully unable to advise you about nutrition and nutritional supplements to help you heal your heart and avoid cardiovascular disease.

Good nutrition is essential for a healthy heart. Your heart never gets to rest. Until the moment of your death, your heart steadily and tirelessly keeps the rhythm of your life. Your heart can only perform this staggering feat if it has an adequate supply of nutrients. To keep your heart pumping strong, feed it the nutrients it needs.

Research conducted at the Center for Health and Wellness and my experience with thousands of patients shows that most heart disease sufferers are deficient in one or more of five key nutrients: CoQ10, L-carnitine, L-arginine, tocopherols, and Vitamin C. The previous chapter described the miracle of CoQ10; this chapter explains the importance of the four additional super-nutrients for your heart.

Who Needs Supplements?

Let's assume you're the ideal patient. You eat your vegetables, you don't smoke, you drink in moderation, you avoid junk food, and you exercise every day. Do you, the role model of healthy living, really need to take vitamins?

In a word, yes. Nutritional supplements help make up for some of the foods we don't eat – and they help compensate for some of the foods we do eat that aren't so good for us. Studies found that people who took a daily multivitamin supplement have stronger immune systems and suffer fewer infections than those who do not take supplements.[1] But there is much more convincing evidence:

- A 1992 US Department of Agriculture study concluded that only 4 percent of the 22,000 Americans studied were getting even the *minimum* recommended daily allowance (RDA) of their essential vitamins.
- A more recent US government survey found that none of the 21,000 people surveyed managed to eat the recommended daily allowance of all the ten basic nutrients studied.[2]
- On any given day, 91 percent of Americans do not consume the recommended amount of fruits and vegetables, with 70 percent not consuming any vitamin-C-rich fruits and 80 percent not consuming any carotene-containing vegetables.
- Today, foods have much less nutritional value than they did a generation ago due to modern methods of agriculture. You would need to eat 60 servings of spinach to get the same amount of iron found in a single serving in 1948!
- In order to get the RDA for vitamin E today, you would need to eat 25 cups of spinach every day. And that may not be enough; several studies have suggested that doses of vitamin E much higher than the RDA may further protect your heart.
- Two-thirds of Americans consume diets deficient in zinc, which is vital for proper immune system functioning.
- Americans often eat the same small number of foods every day, without much variety.

Unless you are the rare exception, you probably don't get even the minimum requirement of all your important vitamins and minerals. These minimum values don't reflect the actual amounts to consume for optimal health.

Nobel laureate Linus Pauling said, "Recommended daily allowances only give levels of vitamins and minerals that will prevent death or serious illness from vitamin deficiency. To get real health benefits from vitamins, you need to get more than the minimal recommended amounts."

Many people have taken multivitamins for years. Vitamin manufacturers now have formulas that include a wide range of antioxidants, which can simplify your routine for heart health.

Store your multivitamin in the refrigerator; the active ingredients stay vital longer. In addition, seeing the vitamin bottle on the shelf next to the orange juice reminds you to take a pill every day.

One more tip: Unless you have iron deficiency, choose a multivitamin without iron. You probably don't need the additional iron. Extra iron can interfere with the absorption of other minerals, give you constipation, and leave a foul taste in your mouth.

Take Healthy Heart Super-Nutrients

While a good multivitamin forms a foundation toward a well-nourished heart, you can further protect your heart with a few additional key nutrients: L-carnitine, L-arginine, tocopherols, and antioxidant doses of vitamin C.

Take L-Carnitine for Energy Plus

L-carnitine plays an essential role in the healthy functioning of the body. Every form of life, from the simplest single-cell organism to the unfathomably complex human body, depends on carnitine for energy production within the cells.

Carnitine shuttles fat (or long-chain fatty acids, to be more precise) into the energy centers or mitochondria of the cells, where the fat can be burned to produce energy. Without enough carnitine, the cell's furnace cannot work at peak efficiency and its energy-production system slows down or stalls. When the body has sufficient carnitine reserves, the cells can burn more fat and generate more energy.

In addition to generating energy, fat burning creates even more health benefits. For example, carnitine-enhanced fat burning prevents the accumulation of excess fat in the heart, liver, and muscles. If allowed to build up, this fat contributes to a number of different health problems, such as heart disease, diabetes, and high triglyceride levels. Carnitine is present in greatest concentrations in the heart, brain, muscles, and testicles, all of which require lots of energy.

Carnitine is often referred to as "the energy vitamin," but it is not really a vitamin at all. A vitamin is a substance that cannot be produced by the body and must be obtained through food. Because the body can synthesize carnitine from the amino acids lysine and methionine, carnitine is not a true vitamin. Other people classify carnitine as an amino acid, but it isn't a true amino acid, either. While carnitine has a chemical structure similar to many amino acids, technically it is a nitrogen-containing, short-chain carboxylic acid. In simple terms, carnitine is a water-soluble, vitamin-like compound similar to the B-complex groups of vitamins.

More than 20 placebo-controlled studies support L-carnitine's role in protecting your heart.[3] Carnitine reduces arterial plaque, lowers LDL cholesterol, and increases HDL levels. These benefits appear in healthy subjects as well as in patients with heart disease.

You obtain carnitine from red meat and dairy. In fact, when scientists first isolated it from the muscle tissue of several animals, they named it carnitine, using the Latin root *carn,* meaning flesh or meat. Unless you eat a diet high in red meat and dairy, it can be difficult to obtain optimal amounts of carnitine from dietary sources alone.

- Take 500 milligrams of L-carnitine as a supplement every day. It is important that you choose the naturally occurring L-carnitine and not the synthetic D,L-carnitine. The D-form interferes with the natural action of the L-carnitine.

Take L-Arginine to Build Heart and Muscles

L-arginine, a naturally occurring amino acid, is the precursor to nitric oxide. L-arginine improves blood flow because in the bloodstream it breaks down into nitric oxide, which helps dilate the blood vessels in the lining of the heart.

Without nitric oxide, your blood vessels narrow. Arterial plaque makes these vessels rigid and restricts blood flow. Recent studies show that arginine supplementation effectively increases the elasticity of blood vessels, providing a much safer alternative to prescription drugs[4]

L-arginine also assists in muscle building. (Remember, the heart is a muscle.) One double-blind study measured the change in muscle strength and lean muscle mass in men taking L-arginine. Men in the study took either L-arginine or a placebo while participating in a strength-training program. Those taking the L-arginine showed a significantly greater increase in muscle strength and lean muscle mass after only five weeks.[5]

Supplements containing L-arginine have been used by athletes for more than 20 years but have become more popular in recent years. Why? Because of the popularity and expense of the prescription drug Viagra. Like arginine, Viagra improves blood flow by increasing nitric oxide levels.

Good food sources of L-arginine include red meat, fish, chicken, beans, chocolate, raisins, nuts, sesame seeds, and sunflower seeds. You can also now find it in supplement form in most nutrition stores.

- Take 500 milligrams of L-arginine daily with food to support muscle growth and heart health. Like carnitine, buy only the L-form of this amino acid.

Take Tocopherols and Tocotrienols to Lower Risks

You may already know that vitamin E helps protect your heart. A number of studies show a link between vitamin E and lowered risk of heart disease. Two landmark studies in the *New England Journal of Medicine* report heart protection from Vitamin E alone. One eight-year study tracked more than 87,000 registered female nurses.[6] A related study followed nearly 40,000 male health care workers.[7] People who took daily vitamin E supplements (100 IU or more) for a minimum of two years had about a 40 percent (41 percent in women, 37 percent in men) lower risk of developing heart disease. They also had a 29 percent lower risk of stroke, and a 13 percent reduction in overall death rates.

This conclusion continues to be supported by the bulk of the evidence but some studies find conflicting results because the supplemental form of vitamin E is a partial solution. New evidence shows that a more natural group of vitamin E-like compounds are more effective.

In nature, vitamin E exists as a mixture of four types of tocopherols and four types of tocotrienols. The vitamin E you find on the drug store shelves contains a single type of tocopherol known as alpha-tocopherol. Taking too much of one tocopherol can block the absorption of the other tocopherols. For this reason, take a blend of both tocopherols and tocotrienols, which is much closer to the way these nutrients exist in nature.

Tocopherols and tocotrienols have many proven health benefits. Tocopherols and tocotrienols fight the free radicals in your body that cause diseases of inflammation (such as rheumatoid arthritis). They also lower your risk of heart disease by increasing your blood circulation, and they lower your risk of cancers of the prostate, colon, and breast.

Many patients have been able to give up their blood-thinning drugs after they begin tocopherol supplementation. There is evidence that a daily supplement of mixed tocopherols increases the elasticity of the arteries.[8] These nutrients also lower risk of heart disease by increasing blood circulation and decreasing the stickiness of platelets in your blood.[9]

You find tocopherols and tocotrienols in "fatty foods," including meat, fish, nuts, oils, dark-green leafy vegetables, seeds, and avocados. However, it is virtually impossible to consume enough of these nutrients in a typical diet. For example, you would have to eat two pounds of sunflower seeds every day to consume all of the tocopherols and tocotrienols you need.

• Take 400 IU of vitamin E with at least 5 milligrams of mixed tocopherols and tocotrienols daily. Vitamin E and the other tocopherols are oil soluble. Like CoQ10, your body can only absorb these nutrients when you eat enough fat. Take them with a teaspoon of almond butter or other natural fat or oil.

Take Vitamin C for Many Benefits

Vitamin C earned a reputation as a preventative for colds since its discovery more than 70 years ago, but it has a lot more to offer. Vitamin C is essential for many of the body's life-sustaining functions. For example, vitamin C:

- fights free radicals;
- helps form collagen (a supportive protein in the tissues);
- sustains the immune system;
- aids in the production of amino acids that regulate the nervous system and
- helps break down histamines which are the inflammatory element of allergic reactions, among many additional functions.

When it comes to cardiovascular disease, studies find a link between low levels of vitamin C and risk of stroke. A 10-year study of more than 2,400 middle-aged men established a relationship between vitamin C intake and reduced risk of stroke.[10] Men with the lowest vitamin C levels had an increased risk of having a stroke 2.4 times greater than men who had higher vitamin C levels. The researchers found that taking vitamin C had more impact on the risk of stroke than being overweight or having high blood pressure.

In addition, researchers at the University of California analyzed the vitamin C intakes and death rates of more than 11,000 men and women.[11] The study showed a dramatic decline in death from heart disease among the men with the highest vitamin C intake, especially among those who took a vitamin C supplement. Merely obtaining the recommended daily allowance for vitamin C through food did not seem to offer any protection against heart disease.

The human body cannot synthesize or produce vitamin C. We can only get this nutrient from our diet – or from supplements. Unfortunately, one-fourth of all Americans do not get even the minimum amount of vitamin C (60 milligrams) that cells need to perform basic biological functions. Foods like oranges, strawberries, broccoli, and bell peppers contain substantial amounts of vitamin C. Still, it is difficult to consume therapeutic amounts of vitamin C from diet alone.

Some drugs, including aspirin, alcohol, analgesics, anti-depressants, anti-coagulants, oral contraceptives, and steroids, reduce the levels of vitamin C in the body. Diabetic and sulfa drugs may not be as effective when taken with large doses of vitamin C. Large doses of vitamin C may cause false negative readings when testing for blood in the stool.

- Take 500 milligrams of vitamin C twice a day with food. At higher doses for shorter periods, vitamin C provides some protection against viruses. If you have a viral illness (such as a cold), take 1000 milligrams every couple of hours with a full glass of water.

Take Extra Antioxidants

Oxygen is essential to life, but at the wrong place at the wrong time, oxygen can damage cells, cause cancer, and contribute to cardiovascular disease and aging through a process known as oxidation. As oxygen makes its way through the body, many of its molecules lose an electron, making them chemically unstable. These ions or free radicals are highly reactive. They strive for stability and ultimately "steal" an electron from another molecule, leaving a damaged molecule in their wake. This oxidative damage can cause changes to DNA, leading to atherosclerosis, as well as cancer, cataracts, arthritis, and many more health problems.

Antioxidants minimize the damage of free radicals by freely donating extra electrons, neutralizing the oxygen molecules before they hurt other cells in the body. Antioxidants include the well-known vitamins A, C, and E, as well as the less famous coenzyme Q10 and lutein, among others. Antioxidants are found in many foods we eat, as well as in nutrition supplements.

Unfortunately, your body's ability to fight free radicals tends to decline with age. In addition, the more active you are – or the "harder you live" – the more likely you are to overwhelm your body's supply of antioxidants. You don't want to stop living hard. Instead, take additional anti-oxidant supplements. After years of research and testing, researchers and doctors have found which antioxidants really work. Earlier in this chapter, you found out about the important antioxidants that are among the super-nutrients for heart health – tocopherols, tocotrienols, and vitamin C. Now let's talk about a few more powerful anti-oxidants that are key to your health.

More Heart-Smart Antioxidants

In addition to the super-nutrients described earlier, many patients take the following heart-smart supplements, too. Not surprisingly, many on the list are antioxidants.

Remember all of the antioxidants (except vitamin C) are oil soluble. That means that the body can only absorb these nutrients when they are in the presence of fat or oil. Take these antioxidants in gel cap form. If possible, look for an "antioxidant supplement," which contains as many of the nutrients as possible in a single pill. Take them with a teaspoon of flaxseed oil or almond butter for best absorption, or take them during a meal with fat.

Alpha Lipoic Acid for energy: Alpha lipoic acid (ALA) plays a vital part in the production of energy in the cells. It earned the name "the universal antioxidant" because of its ability to fight free radicals in both the fatty and watery areas of cells. In addition, ALA recycles and extends the life of other free radicals like vitamin C, E, and CoQ10. ALA lowers the risk of atherosclerosis by fighting specific free radicals that contribute to this disease. Red meat is the best food source of ALA.

• Take 100 milligrams of alpha lipoic acid daily.

Carnosine to support muscles: Carnosine is an important anti-glycation agent that is made from two amino acids naturally present in your nerve and muscle cells. It protects the integrity of the muscle you have, and it helps ensure that new muscle tissue is healthy and long-lasting.

• Take 500 milligrams of carnosine twice a day.

Carotenoids for eyes and immunity: Carotenoids are a family of fat-soluble vitamins with many important benefits for your overall health. They prevent night blindness and free radical damage in your eyes, reducing the risk of developing macular degeneration, the most common cause of blindness in the elderly. Carotenoids also decrease your risk of developing lung and breast cancer. They help support your immune system. Carotenoids are found in meat, milk, eggs, liver, carrots, and spinach.

• Take 2,500 IU of mixed carotenoids daily.

Glutamine for more muscle-building growth hormone: Animal proteins are key food sources of the amino acid glutamine. The human brain contains high concentrations it uses for essential cerebral functions. Glutamine allows the body to increase its levels of growth hormone, making it an important muscle-building supplement. It helps stabilize your energy levels and boosts the natural growth hormone in your body. Growth hormone tells your body to shed fat and build muscle. Glutamine also helps prevent muscle breakdown. Many doctors recommend it to cancer patients to reduce muscle loss. A recent study showed that a glutamine cocktail actually helped people with cancer reverse their muscle loss.[12]

• Take 5 grams of glutamine powder per day. You can dissolve it in water or put it in a protein shake.

Lutein to prevent free radical damage: Lutein is a member of the carotenoid family, and it is a crucial nutrient for eye health. It is one of several carotenoids that make pigment in vegetables; it also contributes to pigment in your retina. Lutein protects vision by neutralizing free radicals in the lens and retina of the eye. It acts like sunglasses by shielding the eye from harmful sunlight. It also lowers the risk of cardiovascular disease and certain cancers by stopping free radical damage that contributes to these diseases. Lutein is in red grapes, egg yolks, squash, peas, and oranges.

• Take 20 milligrams of lutein daily.

Lycopene helps the heart, blood vessels, eyes and more: Lycopene, the pigment found in tomatoes and other red vegetables, is also part of the carotenoid family. Lycopene helps prevent cardiovascular disease by stopping the oxidation of LDH (bad) cholesterol, slowing the buildup of plaque in the arteries. Researchers recently measured the concentrations of lycopene in fat tissue and found that people with higher tissue lycopene levels experienced lower risks of heart attack.[13] It also reduces the risk of prostate and pancreatic cancers by fighting free radical damage. Lycopene also helps prevent macular degeneration by neutralizing free radicals in the eye. Lycopene is found in tomatoes, guava, peppers, watermelon, and pink grapefruit.

- Take 20 milligrams of lycopene daily.

Omega-3 Fatty Acids prevent heart disease and cancer: In the 1970s, some observant scientists noticed that Eskimos eat a lot of fat but have exceptionally low rates of heart disease and cancer. Further study found that the fat in the Eskimo diet was primarily in the form of omega-3 fatty acids, which are found in fatty fish.[14] Over the years, more studies supported the observation that omega-3 fatty acids helps prevent heart disease and cancer.[15]

Omega-3 is one of several essential fatty acids. The omega-3 family includes linolenic, eicosapentaenoic (EPA), and docosahexaenoic (DHA) acids. The body cannot make these acids; you must get them in your diet. Essential fatty acids are necessary for growth and for the overall health of the blood vessels and nerves.

Omega-3s play a central role in protecting the cardiovascular system. Omega-3 fatty acids can calm irregular heart rhythms, lower blood pressure, and lower triglyceride levels.[16] Researchers also found that the cell membranes of heart cells store omega-3s from fish oil to prevent irregular rhythms, which can lead to sudden cardiac death. (Sudden cardiac death is responsible for half of the heart-related deaths in the United States.)

In addition, *The American Journal of Clinical Nutrition* reported a study that shows that fish oil lowers triglyceride levels.[17] The researchers found that participants who took fish oil had a decrease in triglycerides, which reduce their chance of heart disease by 25 percent.

Omega-3 fatty acids also protect against stroke by preventing the formation of sticky blood clots. A recent Harvard study shows that the more men eat foods rich in omega-3 fatty acids, the lower their risk of stroke.[18]

Omega-3 fatty acids are found in cold-water fish, wild game, flaxseed oil, nuts, leafy green vegetable, eggs, and avocados.

- Eat fresh fish two or three times per week.
- Take 3 to 5 grams of omega-3 fish oil a day.

Vitamin A for eyes and more: Vitamin A is a fat-soluble vitamin in the carotenoid family. Vitamin A and beta-carotene are closely related nutrients. Preformed vitamin A (called retinol) is found in animal tissues; beta-carotene is a pigment found in plant foods (especially yellow and orange vegetables and fruits). Because it can be converted to vitamin A in the intestinal tract or liver, beta-carotene is sometimes called provitamin A.

LIVE FAST, GO FAR

An 88-year-old patient who came to the Center for Health and Wellness defied the odds. Despite drinking, smoking, and eating whatever he likes, he's never spent a day in the hospital and he takes no medications. With a quick wit and spring in his step, he could be mistaken for a much younger man. How could this man be so healthy when his health habits were so unhealthy?

With his consent, his doctor performed extensive lab work, and the results were normal in every way but one: He had the highest levels of several key antioxidants they'd ever seen. Since that time, other patients with high levels of antioxidants noticed similar energizing effects. You may experience the same type of rejuvenation by boosting your own levels of antioxidants.

Vitamin A acts as a powerful free radical scavenger, making it a powerful antioxidant. It also prevents night blindness and lowers the risk of developing macular degeneration by preventing free radical damage in the eye. Vitamin A decreases the risk of lung and breast cancer by supporting the immune system. Vitamin A is in meat, milk, eggs, liver, carrots, and spinach.

- Take 2,500 IU of vitamin A daily.

What About All The Other Vitamins?

Does your diet include enough vitamin O? How about vitamin U? Don't worry if these nutrients aren't on your supplement list; they do not exist. This fools a lot of people! It's hard enough to remember all of the genuine vitamins and minerals.

Nutritional supplement manufacturers and distributors contribute to the confusion about many products. Nutritional supplements generate $200 billion in sales each year, and marketers often try to sell you products you just don't need. They use pseudo-science and medical lingo to make it difficult for you to distinguish fact from hype.

At the Center for Health and Wellness, the most commonly asked questions are about nutritional supplementation. Many patients read promotional literature about vitamins and supplements and ask: "Is this stuff for real?"

Separating sound science from the sales pitch can be daunting. Medicine and nutrition are my life's work, yet making sense of this kind of material is still challenging. Too often manufacturers confuse people with scientific-sounding claims that don't make medical sense. For example, some Internet hucksters push "vitamin O," a supplement that claims it will cure arthritis, allergies, asthma, infertility, diabetes, pain, colds, difficulty breathing, obesity, weakened immunity, tumors, lupus, and blood clots, among others. Vitamin O is an outright fraud.

We define a vitamin as a complex, organic substance found in food that is essential for the normal functioning of the human body. The product manufacturer lists the product's "active" ingredient as oxygen. Oxygen isn't organic (it doesn't contain carbon), and it is not a vitamin. A careful reading on the ingredients list – distilled water, sodium chloride (salt), trace minerals, and oxygen molecules – reveals that the product is basically salt water! In this case, the Federal Trade Commission took the manufacturer to court, claiming that the company made unsubstantiated claims. They were forced to pay hundreds of thousands of dollars in restitution.[19]

Products like "vitamin O" make a mockery of nutrition's real role in medicine. Their outrageous claims provide ammunition for the traditional doctors and pharmaceutical companies to insist on a drug-based solution for every health problem.

Unfortunately, vitamin O isn't the only fraud out there. Recently, supplement manufacturers have pushed "vitamin T" (a chemical in sesame seeds said to improve blood disorders) and "vitamin U" (a substance found in cabbage known as S-methyl-methionine, which is said to treat ulcers and tissue damage). Once again, neither vitamin T nor U is a real vitamin.

Your best defense against shysters is knowledge about real vitamins. It not as tough to be informed about vitamins as you might think. Below is a complete list of all the real vitamins with a brief description of what they do and the best food sources.

♥ *Know your real vitamins.*

♥ *Don't believe anything that sounds too good to be true.*

♥ *Look for scientific evidence to back up the claims.*

True Vitamins	Function	Sources
Water Soluble Vitamins		
Vitamin B1 Thiamine	Circulation, blood formation, brain function.	Organ meat, yeast, peas, pork, beans.
Vitamin B2 Riboflavin	Blood cell formation, antibodies, cataract prevention.	Meat, poultry, fish, nuts, kidney, liver, green vegetables.
Vitamin B3 Niacin	Circulation, nervous system, healthy skin	Lean meats, nuts, legumes, potatoes
Vitamin B5 Pantothenic Acid	Adrenal hormones, antibodies, neurotransmitters, stamina.	Eggs, pork, beef, fish, milk, most fruits/vegetables.
Vitamin B6 Pyridoxine	Brain/immune system function, cancer immunity, mild diuretic.	Chicken, fish, kidney, liver, eggs, bananas, lima beans, walnuts.
Vitamin B7 Biotin	Cell growth, metabolism of carbohydrates/fats/proteins.	Liver, eggs yolks, nuts, cauliflower, milk and legumes.
Vitamin B8 Inositol	Hair growth, reduces cholesterol and plaque.	Heart, fruit, milk, nuts, meat and vegetables.
Vitamin B9 Folic Acid	"Brain food", energy, red blood cells, strengthens immunity.	Beef, lamb, pork, chicken liver, eggs, green leafy vegetables, salmon.
Vitamin B12 Cyanocobalamin	Prevent anemia/nerve damage, digestion, cellular longevity.	Lamb, beef, herring, mackerel, pork liver, oysters, poultry, clams, eggs
Vitamin C	Tissue growth/repair, adrenal function, fights cancer/infection.	Citrus, peppers, broccoli, spinach, tomatoes, potatoes, strawberries
Fat Soluble Vitamins		
Vitamin A	Eye problems/skin disorders, healthy bones/teeth, antioxidant.	Liver, fish oil, egg yolks, crab, halibut, whole-milk products; carrots, spinach, broccoli, cantaloupe.
Vitamin D	Absorption of calcium/phosphorus, healthy teeth and bones.	Fish-liver oil, eggs, butter, cream, halibut, herring, liver, mackerel, salmon, sardines, shrimp.
Vitamin E	Prevents cancer, heart disease, cataracts; reduces blood pressure.	Vegetables oils, wheat germ and nuts.
Vitamin K	Produces prothrombin (for blood clotting), healthy liver function.	Green leafy vegetables, dairy prod., eggs, fruits and vegetables.

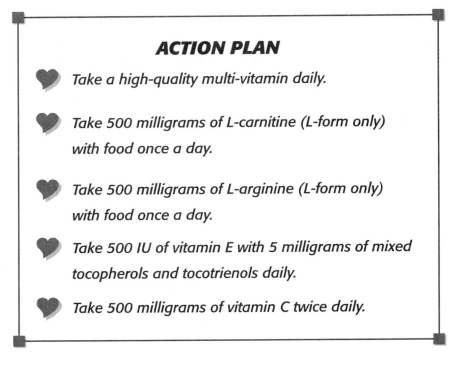

ACTION PLAN

💜 *Take a high-quality multi-vitamin daily.*

💜 *Take 500 milligrams of L-carnitine (L-form only) with food once a day.*

💜 *Take 500 milligrams of L-arginine (L-form only) with food once a day.*

💜 *Take 500 IU of vitamin E with 5 milligrams of mixed tocopherols and tocotrienols daily.*

💜 *Take 500 milligrams of vitamin C twice daily.*

Footnotes Chapter 9

1 Bendich A. Micronutrients in women's health and immune function. *Nutrition.* 2001 Oct; 17(10):858-867.

2 Supplemental Data Tables, USDA Survey, 1994-1996.

3 Borum RP and Bennett SG. Carnitine as an essential nutrient. *Journal of American College of Nutrition.* 1986; 5(2):177-182.

4 *Antioxidant-Amino Acid Mix Shields Blood Vessels,* Reuters Health, 1/22/03.

5 Elam R, Hardin DH, Sutton RA, and Hagen L. Effects of arginine and ornithine on strength, lean body mass and urinary hydroxyproline in adult males. *Journal of Sports Medicine and Physical Fitness,* 1989 Mar; 29(1):52-56.

6 Stampfer MJ, Hennekens CH, Manson JE, et al. Vitamin E consumption and the risk of coronary disease in women. *New England Journal of Medicine.* 1993 May 20; 328(20):1444-1449.

7 Rimm EB, Stampfer MJ, Ascherio A, et al. Vitamin E consumption and the risk of coronary heart disease in men. *New England Journal of Medicine.* 1993 May 20; 328(20):1450-1456.

8 Mottram P, Shige H, and Nestel P. Vitamin E improves arterial compliance in middle-aged men and women. *Atherosclerosis.* 1999 Aug; 145(2):399-404.

9 Mabile L, Bruckdorfer KR and Rice-Evans C. Moderate supplementation with natural alpha-tocopherol decreases platelet aggregation and low-density lipoprotein oxidation. *Atherosclerosis.* 1999 Nov 1; 147(1):177-185.

10 Kurl S, Tuomainen TP, Laukkanen JA, et al. Plasma vitamin C modifies the association between hypertension and risk of stroke. *Stroke.* 2002 Jun; 33(6): 1568-1573.

11 Enstrom JE, Kanim LE and Kleim MA. Vitamin C intake and mortality among a sample of the United States population. *Epidemiology.* 1992 May; 3(3):194-202.

12 May PE, Barber A, D'Olimpio JT, et al. Reversal of cancer-wasting using oral supplementation with a combination of beta-hydroxy-beta-methylbutyrate, arginine and glutamine. *American Journal of Surgery.* 2002 April; 183(4):471-479.

13 Kohlmeier L, Lark JD, Gomez-Gracia E, et al. Lycopene and myocardial infarction risk in the EURAMIC Study. *American Journal of Epidemiology.* 1997 Oct 15; 148(2):618-626.

14 Dyerberg J and Bang HO. Haemostatic function and platelet polyunsaturated fatty acids in Eskimos. *Lancet.* 1979 Sep 1; 2(8140):433-435.

15 Whelton SP, He J, Whelton PK and Muntner P. Meta-analysis of observational studies on fish intake and coronary heart disease. *American Journal of Cardiology.* 2004 May 1; 93(9):1119-1123.

16 Mata Lopez P, et al. Omega-3 fatty acids in the prevention and control of cardiovascular disease. *European Journal of Clinical Nutrition.* 2003 Sep; 57 (Suppl 1):S22-25.

17 Chan DC, Watts GF, Mori TA, et al. Randomized controlled trial of the effect of n-3 fatty acid supplementation on the metabolism of apolipoprotein B-100 and chylomicron remnants in men with visceral obesity. *American Journal of Clinical Nutrition.* 2003 Feb; 77(2):300-307.

18 He K, Rimm EB, Merchant A, et al. Fish consumption and risk of stroke in men. *Journal of the American Medical Association,* 2002 Dec 25; 288(24): 3130-3136.

19 Federal Trade Commission News Release, May 1, 2000.

10

Control the Fire
in Your Heart

You can't feel atherosclerosis or "hardening of the arteries" as it happens. This disease slowly and stealthily forms over the years in response to tiny injuries to the lining of the arteries.

Ironically, the very immune response that keeps you alive causes damage when the injury is to the arteries. Every injury in the body – whether it's a cut on the skin or irritation to the lining of the arteries – triggers the immune system to launch an inflammatory response. Initially, this response speeds the healing of an injured area, but the same white blood cells and inflammatory chemicals that are involved in the health process can also burrow into the artery walls and contribute to heart disease.

The occasional injury to the artery walls heals without major consequences. But chronic injury, year in and year out, results in arteries filled with large patches of plaque build-up, as well as smaller vulnerable plaques filled with inflammatory compounds. At some point, these plaque deposits can erupt and lead to heart attack.

As you might expect, drug companies are hard at work trying to develop drugs to control inflammation and thwart heart disease. Once again, the pharmaceutical companies are misguided. Inflammation is not the enemy; it is the first stage of the healing process. To avoid heart disease, you do not need medication – just avoid the source of the irritation that causes the inflammation in the first place.

In this chapter, you'll discover the link between inflammation and heart disease. You'll also learn about the role of homocysteine in controlling inflammation, and the role of C-reactive protein in detecting it. (For information on testing for homocysteine and C-reactive protein, see Chapter 5, Measure Your Real Heart Health.) In addition, this chapter covers the link between gum disease and cardiovascular disease, including information on what you can do to prevent these problems.

From Inflammation to Heart Attack

A lot of things damage our arteries:

- **Stress hormones:** A sudden spasm in an artery, combined with a surge in stress hormones, may cause the arteries to constrict, resulting in a tiny tear in the endothelium, the lining of the arteries.
- **Hypertension:** People with hypertension may experience blood pressure forces strong enough to injure the delicate arteries.
- **Surgery:** A careless nick or incision in an artery during an angioplasty or other cardiac procedure can damage arteries.
- **Toxins:** A very common cause of arterial damage is toxins in the bloodstream. These irritants – such as cigarette smoke, excess blood glucose or insulin, and oxidized low-density lipoproteins – damage the lining of the arteries as they flow through the bloodstream.

When toxins or traumas injure the arteries, the body triggers an immune response. This process is essentially the same as what happens when you cut yourself shaving or skin your knee. The area typically becomes red, hot, and slightly swollen, all signs that the inflammatory response is working. First, white blood cells, collagen, growth factors, and other chemicals gather to make tissue repairs.

In the arteries, the blood fats (especially harmful LDL cholesterol) rush to the injury site, ultimately adding insult to injury. The LDL cholesterol triggers a cycle of free radical damage. At the same time, white blood cells known as monocytes begin to dig their way into the inner layers of the arteries at the site of the injury. Once they safely enter the artery walls, the white blood cells change into macrophages, or immune cells designed to eat microorganisms and foreign toxins.

At this point, the process of atherosclerosis is well on its way. When the macrophages dine on the oxidized LDL cholesterol pulled from the bloodstream, they change into foam cells, which attract even more cholesterol. The surrounding smooth muscle cells respond by coating the lining of the artery with a layer of collagen and elastin fibers. This leaves you with a layer of arterial plaque, filled with a nasty mixture of dead foam cells, white blood cells, and LDL cholesterol and other fat.

These plaque deposits cause heart attacks in one of two primary ways. Sometimes plaque build-up narrows an artery to the point that it is largely blocked, then a blood clot loosens and lodges in one of these restricted arteries. Other times smaller plaque lesions rupture and cause heart attacks. When these lesions burst – perhaps in response to a sudden rise in blood pressure or heartbeat – they dump their contents into the artery, immediately attracting another round of clotting factors and inflammatory chemicals. If a thrombus, or blood clot, blocks your coronary artery, you have a heart attack.

Reduce Homocysteine Easily

In 1968, the deaths of an eight-year-old boy and a two-month-old infant from massive strokes caught the attention of a Boston pathologist named Kilmer McCully. In examining the cases, McCully noticed that both children had a genetic defect in the way their bodies handled homocysteine, a metabolic by-product of eating protein and a major cause of inflammation in the blood vessels. As a result of this inherited problem, both children had cholesterol-clogged and damaged arteries. McCully made the connection between the high levels of homocysteine in the blood and the cardiovascular disease in the kids.[1]

For years, other doctors mocked McCully, but now experts recognize high homocysteine levels as a major risk factor for cardiovascular disease. In fact, according to a 1997 study, "An increased plasma total homocysteine level confers an independent risk of vascular disease similar to that of smoking or hyperlipidemia (high levels of fats in the blood)."[2] It all boils down to this: If you have elevated levels of homocysteine in your blood, you are three times more likely to have a heart attack than someone with normal homocysteine, regardless of your cholesterol levels.

Homocysteine is a toxic amino acid that irritates the lining of the blood vessels, causing inflammation and cardiovascular disease. When you have too much homocysteine in your blood, your blood vessels cannot dilate properly, which can cause problems in times of stress. Inadequate blood flow to the heart can cause heart attacks; inadequate blood flow to the brain can cause strokes.

The link between homocysteine levels and cardiovascular disease is unmistakable. In all, at least 20 studies showed strong links between homocysteine and devastating cardiac events, including a landmark report that tracked 15,000 male physicians in the Physician's Health Study.[3] This study found participants with high homocysteine levels were three times as likely to have a heart attack, regardless of their cholesterol levels. Taken together, the research shows that homocysteine levels predict cardiovascular events better than cholesterol levels.

Despite these findings, however, many patients have never heard of homocysteine. One reason the public remains relatively uninformed about this risk factor is that no big drug companies market drugs to reduce homocysteine levels. If Pfizer made a drug to treat high homocysteine, it would be a household word.

Drug companies haven't tried to market homocysteine-lowering drugs because you don't need them. B vitamins help the body breakdown homocysteine. All patients at the Center for Health and Wellness lowered their elevated homocysteine levels with nothing more than a vitamin supplement.

Measure Inflammation with C-Reactive Protein

Twenty-five million Americans are in danger of suffering a heart attack and don't know it. Are you among them? Find out if you are at risk by having a simple blood test for C-reactive protein, or CRP.

C-reactive protein (CRP) was recently recognized as an excellent predictor of heart disease. When part of your body is injured, it sends out signals asking for help. The immune system responds by sending white blood cells and inflammatory molecules (including CRP) to the injured area.

These defense cells try to fix the injured areas and fight off any intruders, but this defensive response causes inflammation. The inflammatory response requires energy in the form of oxidative "fire" that can damage surrounding tissues. Inflammation of blood vessel cells is the major process leading to heart disease.

Elevated CRP levels indicate that there is inflammation in the body. Using this measure, we can detect hidden heart disease using CRP better than with cholesterol levels. The *New England Journal of Medicine* recently published a study on CRP that involved nearly 28,000 participants. Researchers tried to predict cardiac events (heart attack and stroke) using LDL cholesterol and CRP levels in the blood. They found that CRP predicted cardiac events better than LDL cholesterol did.[4]

What can you do to keep your levels of CRP low? The best way is with exercise. We recently discovered that even moderate physical activity can lower CRP levels. People who went from not exercising at all to exercising a small amount five times a week cut their CRP levels by as much as 30 percent.[5]

Several supplements also help stop cell damage and irritation in your heart's lining. By avoiding damage to your heart, you can lower your CRP level and lower your risk of a heart attack. These heart-saving supplements include L-arginine, folic acid, taurine, vitamin E, and vitamin C. You'll find out more how you can use them to improve your cardiac health in this chapter. You may remember the information about having your CRP levels tested from reading Chapter 5, Measure Your Real Heart Health.

Prevent Heart Disease With a Healthy Smile

Good dental hygiene gives you more than a winning smile and fresh breath; it gives you a healthier heart as well. Studies found that people with gum disease suffer heart attacks more often than those with healthy gums and teeth.[6] A major study by the US Department of Veterans Affairs found that men with severe periodontal bone loss had 150 percent greater risk of heart disease.[7] An even larger study, known as the Arteriosclerosis Risk in Communities Study, found that people with gum disease have a 1.5 fold increase rate of heart disease.[8]

The problem begins when plaque forms on your teeth. Bacteria forms dental plaque, causing tooth decay and creating inflammation and infection of the surrounding tissues. The infection destroys the fibers and bone that hold the teeth and gums in place. The gums separate from the teeth, creating more spaces for plaque to form and bacteria to breed. Over time, these pockets deepen and destroy the gum tissue and bone. Eventually your teeth migrate out of place or even loosen and fall out.

This condition poses a serious threat to your cardiovascular health. The bacteria in your mouth can sneak through diseased gums and enter the bloodstream, where they cause inflammation. In the bloodstream, the bacteria travel throughout the body and trigger an immune response.

The chronic infection activates the white blood cells, which can cause arterial lesions and encourage plaque build-up on the walls of your arteries. These arterial plaque deposits thicken and narrow the walls of the artery. This decreases blood flow to the heart and brain, increasing your risk of heart attack and stroke.

University of Michigan researchers found periodontal bacteria in the fatty deposits in the linings of the blood vessels of patients with periodontal as well as cardiovascular disease.[9]

Not surprisingly, people with gum disease also have elevated levels of C-reactive protein, putting them at risk for heart disease. A ground-breaking study conducted in 1997 by the University of North Carolina at Chapel Hill first linked high C-reactive protein levels with patients who had gum disease.[10] More studies confirmed this finding. Research at the University of Buffalo found that people with diseased gums had significantly higher levels of bacterial inflammatory components in their bloodstream.[11] Interestingly, additional studies show that CRP levels drop when the gum disease is treated.

According to the Academy of General Dentistry, more than half of American men have some form of gum disease. Many medications can actually make your gum problems worse. For example, diuretics used to treat high blood pressure can reduce saliva production, which increases plaque buildup. Calcium channel blockers such as Procardia and Cardizem can enlarge your gums, making it more difficult for you to clean your teeth and gums effectively. Cholesterol-lowering statin drugs block the best treatment for gum disease, coenzyme Q10. If you are taking any of these drugs, talk to your doctor about safer alternatives.

Prevent Gum Disease

Fortunately, you can prevent or reverse gum disease. First, you must practice good oral hygiene.

To get your teeth sparkling clean, start by brushing your teeth for a full three to four minutes at least twice a day. Most people brush for less than half the time – and most of us fail to floss, although it has been established that flossing helps clean between the teeth. Be sure to clean along the gum line. That's where damaging plaque hides. Floss once a day to get the plaque that forms between the teeth the brushing can't reach.

Get professional cleanings regularly. If your teeth and gums are healthy, twice a year is adequate. If you have problems with plaque and hard deposits (tartar), you may need to visit the dentist more often. Maintaining healthy gums and teeth won't only save your smile, it may help to save your life.

THE ANTIOXIDANT ANSWER

In addition to regular brushing and flossing, a daily dose of antioxidants helps protect your smile. You read about the benefit of many of these antioxidants for your heart. Here are recommendations to help your gums as well:

- Take vitamin C: This hard-working antioxidant helps reduce the inflammation associated with gingivitis. It also repairs the connective tissues of your gums. Take 500 milligrams twice a day.
- Take coenzyme Q10: This powerful antioxidant can reverse gum disease and reduce your risk of heart attack at the same time. To prevent gum disease, take 60 milligrams once a day. To treat existing gum disease, take 100 milligrams twice a day.
- Take folic acid: This nutrient helps regenerate damaged gum tissue. Oral rinses containing folic acid can be effective in treating gum disease.[12] You may need to contact a holistic dentist in your area.

- Take vitamin E: Take 400 IU daily as part of a high-quality multivitamin.
- Take zinc: This mineral helps protect and heals gum tissues. Take 30 milligrams daily.

ACTION PLAN

Take B vitamins to lower your homocysteine levels.

Recommended dosages:

 25 milligrams of vitamin B2

 25 milligrams of vitamin B6

 500 micrograms of vitamin B12

 800 micrograms of folate

Visit your dentist every six months. Brush twice a day, and floss once a day.

Take antioxidants to improve the health of your gums:

Recommended dosages:

 Vitamin C: 500 milligrams twice a day

 Coenzyme Q10: 100 milligrams twice a day (if you have gum disease)

 Vitamin E: 400 IU daily

 Zinc: 30 milligrams daily

Footnotes Chapter 10

1 McCully KS. Homocysteine, vitamins and prevention of vascular disease. *Military Medicine.* 2004 Apr; 169(4):325-329.

2 Graham IM, Daly LE, Refsum HM, et al. Plasma homocysteine as a risk factor for vascular disease: The European Concerted Action Project. *Journal of the American Medical Association.* 1997 Jun 22; 277(22):1775-1781.

3 Chasan-Taaber L, Shelhub J, Rosenberg IH, et al. A prospective study of folate and vitamin B6 and risk of myocardial infarction in US physicians. *Journal of the American College of Nutrition.* 1996 Apr; 15(2):136-143.

4 Ridker P, Rifai N, Rose L, et al. Comparison of C-reactive protein and low-density lipoprotein cholesterol levels in the predication of first cardiovascular events. *New England Journal of Medicine.* 2002 Nov 14; 347(20):1557-1565.

5 Church T, Barlow CE, Earnest CP, et al. Association between cardiorespiratory fitness and C-reactive protein in men. Arteriosclerosis and Thrombosis: *Journal of Vascular Biology.* 2002 Nov 1; 22(11):1869-1879.

6 Genco R. Periodontal disease and cardiovascular disease: epidemiology and possible mechanisms. *Journal of American Dental Association.* 2002 Jun; 133 Supple: 14S-22S.

7 Beck J, Garcia R, Heiss G, et al. Periodontal disease and Cardiovascular disease. *Journal of Periodontistry.* 1996 Oct; 67(10 Suppl):1123-1137.

8 Kilgore C. Periodontitis and Independent Risk Factor for Coronary Heart Disease. *Family Practice News,* Aug. 01, 2000.

9 Clarkson BH. The Link Between Systemic Conditions and Diseases and Oral Health. University of Michigan – Ann Arbor. *Abstract of Presentation at AAAS Annual Meeting:* January 22, 1999.

10 Williamson D. New Research Finds Link Between Gum Disease, Acute Heart Attacks. University of North Carolina at Chapel Hill, Nov 8, 2000.

11 Genco RJ. UB Researchers Identify Specific Oral Bacteria Most Likely to Increase Risk of Heart Attack. University of Buffalo, Mar 12, 1999.

12 Pack AR. Folate mouthwash: effects on established gingivitis in periodontal patients. *Journal of Clinical Periodontology.* 1984 Oct; 11(9):619-628.

11

Individualize
Your Doctor's Heart Cure

Heart disease rarely occurs spontaneously. It usually strikes in response to other ongoing health problems. You could have these other conditions for years or even decades before evidence of heart disease surfaces. To prevent or reverse heart disease and promote overall health, it's important to address these underlying conditions.

While *The Doctor's Heart Cure's* core program applies to everyone, this chapter can help you adapt this approach to your individual situation. Specifically, you'll find natural methods to reverse high blood pressure, diabetes, obesity, and chronic muscle loss. One or more of these problems usually precede or co-exist with heart disease. Your *Doctor's Heart Cure* program will be incomplete if you don't reverse these problems as well.

In addition, although cholesterol is not a major cause of heart disease, heart disease and cholesterol problems often occur together. If you have heart disease and an unhealthy cholesterol profile, this chapter will help you develop a plan to improve your cholesterol levels without depending on harmful prescription drugs. In this chapter, if you tested low in lean body mass, you'll also find a clinically tested program for building muscle where it counts.

Lower Your High Blood Pressure

If you have hypertension, your body is telling you something. Hypertension – or high blood pressure – is more than a medical annoyance.

It's a warning sign that you may face heart disease with all its consequences if you do not take steps to control it.

The high pressure in your blood vessels can damage the delicate tissues of your eyes, kidney and brain. It often leads to heart attacks, strokes, loss of vision, and kidney failure. In fact, people with hypertension face a risk of heart attack three times greater and a risk of stroke seven times greater than that of people with normal blood pressure.

High blood pressure is very common. About one out of ten Americans have it and your risk gradually goes up with age. More than half of all elderly Americans have unhealthy high blood pressure. You are at higher risk if you are African American, smoke, are overweight, or have a family history of hypertension. Fortunately, it's very likely that you can lower your blood pressure by making slight changes in your diet and lifestyle.

HEED THE WARNING SIGNS

We call hypertension "the silent killer" because it strikes without warning. Unfortunately, about 20 percent of Americans with high blood pressure don't know they have the condition, and only one-third do something about it. Advanced hypertension can sometimes cause headaches (especially in the morning), fatigue, dizziness, rapid pulse, shortness of breath, sweating, nosebleeds, and visual problems. The only way to be sure your blood pressure is under control is to have your blood pressure checked.

Follow these simple and effective measures to prevent or reverse high your blood pressure:

- Don't smoke. Nicotine produces drug-like actions directly on your heart and blood vessels. It constricts arteries and thereby elevates blood pressure and increases the work done by your heart. If you have high blood pressure and you smoke, you are five times more likely to have a heart attack and sixteen times more likely to have a stroke than if you don't smoke.

- Lose weight, if necessary. People who carry extra weight tend to have high blood pressure. About half of all people with hypertension are overweight. An analysis of five studies involving weight loss and hypertension found that, on average, losing 20 pounds resulted in a decline of 6.3 mm Hg in systolic and 3.1 mm Hg in diastolic pressure.
- Avoid certain over-the-counter medicines. Avoid using antihistamines, decongestants, cold remedies, and appetite suppressants, because these medications tend to raise blood pressure.
- Avoid excess coffee and caffeinated beverages, which can elevate blood pressure. Limit coffee to one or two cups in the morning.
- Limit alcohol consumption. While there are heart benefits with modest drinking, consuming more than 30 milliliters of alcohol a day – an amount equal to one ounce of 100-proof whiskey, 8 ounces of wine, or two 12-ounce beers – can raise your blood pressure.
- Learn techniques to relax. Stress leads to the excess secretion of cortisol. A prolonged increase in cortisol leads to negative health conditions including high blood pressure. Meditation and relaxation techniques are good ways to lower your stress and improve your health.
- Use PACE™ exercises on a regular schedule to strengthen your cardio-respiratory capacity as described in Chapter 7. These exercises also help reduce your resting blood pressure.

Let Thy Food be Thy Blood Pressure Medicine

- **Use Cayenne Peppers:** Cayenne contains a compound called capsaicin, a mild blood thinner that reduces platelet stickiness. Generally, the hotter the pepper, the more capsaicin it contains. Other constituents of cayenne are vitamin E and vitamin C. Research shows cayenne can help you improve circulation, fight inflammation, clear congestion, boost immunity, and lose weight.
  - Eat hot peppers to your taste.

- **Snack on celery:** Eating celery (as well as consuming celery oil and celery seeds) helps to lower blood pressure by relaxing the smooth muscles in the blood vessels. Chomping on as few as four stalks of celery a day provides enough of the active ingredient, a compound known as 3-butylphthalide, to reduce blood pressure.

- Eat four stalks of celery daily.

- **Go heavy on the garlic:** Garlic is very effective at lowering high blood pressure. It is a natural vasodilator (it widens blood vessels). Studies find garlic lowers systolic pressure by an impressive 20 to 30 mm Hg and diastolic by 10 to 20 mm Hg. A 12-week German study shows powdered garlic aided significantly in lowering blood pressure. The study documented another finding: garlic produced a significant drop in cholesterol and triglycerides in the test subjects.[1]
  - If your blood pressure is high, try adding garlic to every meal. That's not hard to do once you get in the habit. You can also peel off the outer layer and eat a raw clove of garlic daily. If you prefer to use a supplement, look for a product that contains at least 3,600 micrograms of allicin, the active ingredient, per dose.

- **Maintain an optimum potassium level for heart health.** Low potassium level may cause heart disease. Choosing the right foods is the best way to ensure you're getting enough potassium, particularly after exercise. The widespread use of diuretics (water pills) prescribed for high blood pressure often cause low potassium levels. ACE inhibitors and beta-blockers also impair potassium levels. In addition, modern food processing and increased sodium levels can cause your potassium levels to drop.

  The most common symptoms of low potassium are muscle cramps and weakness, accompanied by thirst and frequent urination. Diets low in potassium often precede high blood pressure! The best way to get potassium is from food, not supplements. Most nuts and many fruit provide potassium. See the following table for your best sources.

Food	Potassium
Figs (10 pieces, dried)	1,352 mg
Avocado (whole or 1 cup)	1,319 mg
Sun Dried Tomatoes (1/2 cup)	1,272 mg
Pistachios (1 cup)	1,241 mg
Apricots (1 cup)	1,222 mg
Winter Squash (1 cup, mashed)	1,070 mg
Almonds (1 cup, unsalted)	1,039 mg
Pumpkin Kernels (1/2 cup)	945 mg
Bananas (1 large)	467 mg

- Maintain optimum levels of calcium and magnesium for heart health. Low levels of calcium and magnesium can contribute to hypertension. Fortunately, it's easy to use either dietary changes or supplements to increase your calcium and magnesium. Rich dietary sources to help reverse the condition include dairy, small fish and nuts.

Calcium Rich Foods	Magnesium Rich Foods
Milk (1 cup)	Almonds (1/3 cup)
Yoghurt (1 cup)	Tofu (1/2 cup)
Salmon (3 ounces)	Cashews (1 cup)
Cheese (1 ounce)	Raisin Bran (1/3 cup)

Use Nutritional Supplements to Lower Your Blood Pressure

- **Take Coenzyme Q10:** Our Wellness Research Foundation has found that most people with high blood pressure have CoQ10 levels far below the therapeutic range. We have also found that virtually all patients are successful at achieving therapeutic blood levels by taking an oral CoQ10 supplement. Most importantly, more than half of the patients who come to the Center for Health and Wellness with high blood pressure already take blood pressure drugs from another doctor have been able to wean themselves from those drugs using CoQ10.

- Take 100 milligrams of CoQ10 daily and ask your doctor to measure the CoQ10 in your blood.

- **Calcium and magnesium:** If you find you can't get sufficient calcium or magnesium through diet, then supplements may be in order.
  - Take 500 milligrams of calcium and 500 milligrams of magnesium daily.

- **Use vitamin C:** A major ten-year study showed that the lower the levels of vitamin C, the higher a person's blood pressure and risk of stroke.[2] One study found that taking as little as 250 milligrams of vitamin C a day slashed the risk of high blood pressure by almost half.[3]
  - Take 1,000 milligrams of vitamin C daily.

Lower Your Blood Pressure with Herbs

Again, if your blood pressure is not improved with foods alone or supplements then use one or more of the remedies listed below. Do not use herbs in place of good nutrition. You can find these herbs at most health food stores.

- **Use astralagus:** Chinese and Indian herbalists have used astralagus to treat heart disease for centuries. It contains numerous minerals, amino acids, and flavonoids, some of which are credited with its blood-pressure lowering powers.
  - Take 500 milligrams of powdered astralagus root in capsule form twice a day. If you prefer liquid extract form, take 5 milliliters (one teaspoon) twice a day.

- **Use dandelion:** Dandelion is a natural diuretic and an excellent alternative to water pills. Yes, the weed that invades your lawn each summer produces a mild water-elimination effect (but not enough to produce dehydration). Dandelion leaves also contain vitamins and minerals, including vitamins A, C, D, potassium, and calcium.

  • Take 250 milligrams of dandelion two or three times a day.

• **Use cat's claw:** This South American vine is a natural diuretic indigenous Amazonians use. Its name comes from its claw-like thorns. Athletes often use it to lose water weight before a competition. Its effect is gentle.

  • Take 500 milligrams of cat's claw twice a day, until it eliminates the excess fluid.

• **Use hawthorn:** Widely used in Europe, hawthorn lowers blood pressure, improves coronary (blood vessels that supply the heart itself) circulation, prevents cholesterol deposits from forming on artery walls, and helps strengthen the heart muscle. It works as a natural beta blocker, allowing the arteries to open so blood flows freely. In a recent 10-week study, hawthorn extract produced a significant therapeutic reduction in diastolic blood pressure. Hawthorn also reduced anxiety better than magnesium or a placebo.[4]

  • Take 500 milligrams of hawthorn extract, with food, twice a day.

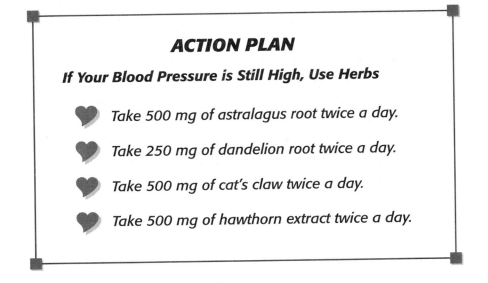

ACTION PLAN

If Your Blood Pressure is Still High, Use Herbs

💜 *Take 500 mg of astralagus root twice a day.*

💜 *Take 250 mg of dandelion root twice a day.*

💜 *Take 500 mg of cat's claw twice a day.*

💜 *Take 500 mg of hawthorn extract twice a day.*

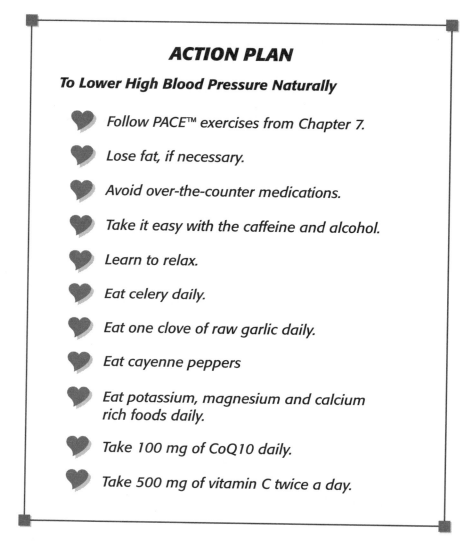

ACTION PLAN

To Lower High Blood Pressure Naturally

- Follow PACE™ exercises from Chapter 7.
- Lose fat, if necessary.
- Avoid over-the-counter medications.
- Take it easy with the caffeine and alcohol.
- Learn to relax.
- Eat celery daily.
- Eat one clove of raw garlic daily.
- Eat cayenne peppers
- Eat potassium, magnesium and calcium rich foods daily.
- Take 100 mg of CoQ10 daily.
- Take 500 mg of vitamin C twice a day.

Improve Your Cholesterol Profile

Remember the VAP cholesterol test that from Chapter 5? It is more effective in predicting heart attack or stroke than the usual cholesterol test and identifies 90 percent of cholesterol problems. Don't rely on tests that only tell you your total cholesterol or LDL are high. With cholesterol, ferreting out the details can guide you to crucial improvements.

You may not really need to lower your total cholesterol, but if you are like most Americans, you may need to improve other cholesterol parameters. The most important and the most likely to need improvement is HDL cholesterol. HDL cholesterol is the most beneficial of cholesterols and is protective against heart disease. Exercise is by far the most effective tool to increase your HDL cholesterol. What kind of exercise boosts HDL the most? Interval training.

Remember from Chapter 2 that interval training also protects you from heart disease by building reserve heart and lung capacity. A typical PACE™ program takes only about 15 minutes a day. This, not diet, is the most important single action you can take to manage your cholesterol. You will find advice you can use to build your own program in Chapter 7, Build Heart Strength. In this section, you will find natural remedies to use with interval exercises to improve your cholesterol ratios.

Choose Food to Improve Your Cholesterol

- **Make protein a high priority:** In Chapter 6, you learned about a plan for eating and enjoying real food – a good-fat, good-protein, good-fruits and vegetables diet. Each of the three basic types of food – protein, fat, and carbohydrates – induces a different hormonal response. When you eat protein, your body produces growth hormones that build muscles. When you eat carbohydrates, your body secretes insulin to digest them and build fat. Eating fat has a neutral hormonal response.

  Remember, over the long haul, low-fat diets are counter-productive to health. When you eat a low-fat diet, you not only eat more carbohydrates but you also inadvertently sacrifice the most important nutrient, protein. If you follow the low-fat advice, you will lose vital muscle – including heart muscle – and burden your heart with flab.

  Therefore, eat plenty of protein and the right kinds of fat, and keep your carbohydrate intake low. This allows you to lose body fat, control carbohydrate cravings, and keep your cholesterol levels healthy.

- **Eat Olives and Use Olive Oil:** Eating olives lowers your cholesterol, your risk of heart disease and can help prevent cancer. Whole olives have a high proportion of essential amino acids and are high in vitamins E, K, and A. The vitamin E in olives prevents oxidative stress caused by things like pollution, sunlight and cigarette smoke.

  The USDA named green olives as the second best source for Vitamin K, which your body needs for proper bone formation, blood clotting and cancer prevention.[5]

  Both olives and olive oil contain monounsaturated fats. These good fats lower LDL and raise HDL cholesterol levels. They also prevent the build-up of plaque on your artery walls.

  Olives are great at satisfying hunger without consuming lots of food. One large California olive has fewer then seven calories. The intensity of flavor in olives makes a little go a long way.

  - Use olive oil in cooking and on salads.
  - Try olives for flavoring dishes and as snacks.

- **Eat plant sterols:** The July 2003 issue of the *Journal of the American Medical Association* compared the cholesterol-lowering properties of three diets. In this study, the first group of people ate a "control diet" very low in saturated fat. The second group took the statin drug Lovastatin. The third group ate a diet high in plant sterols, fiber, and almonds. Those in the first group who ate low-fat diet decreased their cholesterol by only 8 percent, and decreased C-reactive protein levels by 10 percent. Those in the second group who took statin drug decreased cholesterol levels by 30 percent and C-reactive protein levels, 33 percent. The third group of people who ate a diet high in plant sterols decreased their cholesterol by 29 percent and C-reactive protein by 28 percent.[6]

  The statins and plant sterols worked equally well for those in the second and third groups. Stated another way, the plant sterol diet provides the cardiovascular benefits without the harmful side effects associated with the prescription drugs. The side effects associated with Lovastatin include liver toxicity, weakness and fatigue, bursting muscle fibers, CoQ10 inhibition, and kidney failure. There are no negative side effects to following the plant sterol diet.

You can easily include natural sources of plant sterols in your diet by eating nuts and vegetables.[7] Plants with nutritious sterols also have the fats that are good for the heart. Add these foods to your diet: Almonds, eggplant, eggs, flaxseed, fresh fruit, okra, olive oil, olives, and walnuts.

- Eat a diet high in plant sterols.

- **Use fiber:** A high-fiber diet helps lower cholesterol levels. The average American consumes only 11 grams of fiber a day, far short of the 25 grams recommended. If you don't care for high-fiber foods, take a psyllium-based supplement, following package directions. One study found that people who took one tablespoon of a soluble-fiber supplement twice a day for eight weeks had a 7 percent reduction in their low-density lipoprotein (LDL) levels.[8]
  - Eat high-fiber foods. If necessary, take a psyllium-based supplement daily, following package directions.

- **Eat Garlic:** Garlic, a member of the onion and leek family, lowers cholesterol levels, inhibits blood clots, thins the blood, and dilates blood vessels.
  - Eat one to three cloves of garlic daily.

- **Eat Foods High in Omega-3 Fatty Acids:** Omega-3s play a central role in protecting your cardiovascular system. The cell membranes of heart cells store omega-3 from fish oil. This storage prevents irregular rhythms, which can lead to sudden cardiac death (SCD). SCD is responsible for half of the heart-related deaths in the United States.
  - Fish oil lowers triglyceride levels in your blood linked to heart disease. Patients taking the fish oil had a decrease in triglycerides which reduced their chance of heart disease by 25.[9] Increase your omega-3 fatty acid intake with fish oils, avocados, nuts, olives and eggs.

Use Nutrition to Lower your Cholesterol

- **Policosanol:** This organic plant alcohol lowers "bad" cholesterol without harmful side effects.
  - Take 20 milligrams of policosanol daily.

- **Take niacin:** This vitamin plays an active role in more than fifteen metabolic reactions, most of which give you energy from carbohydrates. Niacin lowers LDL (bad) cholesterol and triglycerides while raising HDL (good) cholesterol. It also improves circulation by dilating the blood vessels.
  - Take 50 milligrams of niacin daily.

- **Take vitamin C:** This vitamin is essential for cholesterol metabolism. It is responsible for the excretion of excess cholesterol from the body.
  - If you have unhealthy cholesterol, increase your Vitamin C to 1500 mgs twice a day.

- **Take vitamin E:** This antioxidant helps prevent free radical damage, in addition to helping the body maintain cardiac and smooth muscle. It also keeps one particular form of LDL cholesterol from oxidizing and forming plaque deposits on the arteries.
  - Take 400 IU of vitamin E with mixed tocopherols and tocotrienols daily.

- **Carnitine:** Carnitine is necessary for fat burning and energy production in every one of your cells. It brings fatty acids to the mitochondria of your cells where they produce energy. Your heart muscle has the highest energy requirements. That is why it is particularly vulnerable to carnitine deficiencies.
Carnitine's benefits also include reducing arterial plaque, lowering LDL cholesterol and increasing HDL levels.
You can get carnitine from red meat and dairy. But it is hard to get enough from your daily diet. It is important that you choose the naturally occurring L-carnitine and not the synthetic D,L-carnitine. The D

form interferes with the action of the L-carnitine.
- Take 500mg Carnitine each day.

- **CoQ10:** Once again, studies show this energizing nutrient effectively and safely lowers cholesterol. It provides energy for the heart, lowers cholesterol, and blood pressure. CoQ10 is the single most important heart nutrient that you can take.
  - Take 100 milligrams of CoQ10 per day and ask your doctor to check your blood level.

Use Herbs to Improve Cholesterol

- **Use ginger:** This root, which is native to tropic and semi-tropic regions, lowers and stops oxidation of cholesterol. It also acts as a blood thinner. A study in *The Journal of Nutrition* proved that ginger lowers cholesterol. Mice with high cholesterol took ginger extract for 10 weeks. The mice that took the ginger had significantly lower cholesterol.[10]
  - Take 300 milligrams of ginger twice daily.

- **Use gugulipid:** Hindu medicine has used gugulipid, an extract from the Guggal tree, for centuries to lower cholesterol. In 1987, India approved gugulipid as a treatment for obesity and lipid disorders. Recent research published in the journal *Annual Review of Nutrition* shows that gugulipid blocks receptors that manage cholesterol levels, allowing the body to remove more cholesterol from the bloodstream.[11]
  - Take 20 milligrams of gugulipid daily.

- **Use cinnamon:** Eating 1/2 teaspoon of cinnamon daily can lower blood sugar, triglycerides, LDL cholesterol, and total cholesterol. Cinnamon contains a chemical that helps cells recognize and respond to insulin.
  - Try adding a dash of cinnamon to your morning cup of coffee.

ACTION PLAN

To Improve Cholesterol

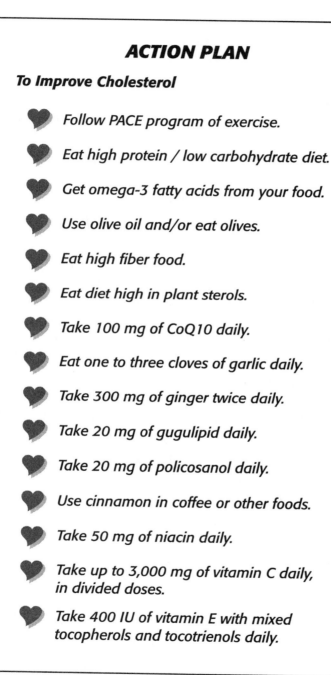

Follow PACE program of exercise.

Eat high protein / low carbohydrate diet.

Get omega-3 fatty acids from your food.

Use olive oil and/or eat olives.

Eat high fiber food.

Eat diet high in plant sterols.

Take 100 mg of CoQ10 daily.

Eat one to three cloves of garlic daily.

Take 300 mg of ginger twice daily.

Take 20 mg of gugulipid daily.

Take 20 mg of policosanol daily.

Use cinnamon in coffee or other foods.

Take 50 mg of niacin daily.

Take up to 3,000 mg of vitamin C daily, in divided doses.

Take 400 IU of vitamin E with mixed tocopherols and tocotrienols daily.

Reverse Diabetes

A few years ago a new patient, Will, a middle-aged African-American man with diabetes and high blood pressure, came to the Center for Health and Wellness. He took several prescription medications and injected himself with insulin for years. Will's doctor insisted he would have to take insulin shots for the rest of his life. He told Will that genetics caused his diabetes because his mother also had diabetes.

Will delivered mail for a living and worked out at the gym regularly so he was not overly sedentary. He said, "I'm eating healthy. I follow all the recommendations." But as Will talked more, it was clear that the advice he had been given was to eat a low-fat diet. This is the advice most diabetics receive and is amazingly, the dietary advice of the American Diabetic Association. This is exactly the wrong advice for a diabetic. Fat in the diet does not cause diabetes, starches do. What's more, when you eat low-fat you will eat more of the real culprit – starches. Will followed the advice of his doctor and the American Diabetic Association by avoiding sugar and fat, but not starches. In fact, he ate starches at every meal: cereal for breakfast, pasta for lunch, and potatoes and bread with dinner.

Will was surprised to learn that his body converts all those starches he eats into sugars in his body, flooding his bloodstream with glucose. Will switched to a diet of foods low on the glycemic index, and added several herbs and nutritional supplements. In several months, he no longer needed insulin shots; he has not taken insulin in several years now and has no signs of diabetes.

How could Will overcome his genetic inheritance? When he severely restricted his carbohydrates for a time, his insulin levels declined and his insulin receptor switches reset to their "pre-diabetic" setting. The Center for Health and Wellness has treated hundreds of patients like Will, and by following this approach these people were able to overcome their diabetes. Begin by following the eating recommendations in Chapter 6. Then, if you have diabetes, add the tips that follow in this chapter.

Eat Better to Beat Diabetes

To reverse diabetes, follow the high protein, low carbohydrate diet described in Chapter 6 and the PACE™ exercise in Chapter 7.

- **Grassfed Beef:** The old saying "you are what you eat" is true. Commercial beef has drastically less nutritional value than their pasture-fed relatives do. A study in the November 2000 issue of the *Journal of Animal Science* found that the more grass cattle ate, the more nutritious their beef became.[12]

  Grassfed products have three to five times more conjugated linoleic acid (CLA) than that of commercial animals.[13] CLA is an important nutrient that has cancer-preventing properties. Grassfed beef also has 4 times more Vitamin E.[14]

- **Use fiber:** Soluble fiber helps stabilize blood sugar. To help control glucose levels, eat a diet rich in soluble fiber. Soluble fiber supplements are also available from health food stores.
  - Eat a diet rich in soluble fiber.

- **Use garlic:** This herb helps lower blood-sugar levels.
  - Eat up to three cloves of garlic daily, or use a commercially prepared product.

- **Almonds:** Almonds have been shown to help people lose weight and reduce the need for type 2 diabetes medicine. Fully 96 percent of the patients in a recent study were able to reduce their need for medication.[15]
  - Eat almonds as snacks whenever you like.

Use Nutrition to Reverse Diabetes

- **Use chromium:** Studies find that people with adult-onset diabetes can lower their insulin requirements by taking chromium supplements. Chromium makes insulin about ten times more efficient at processing sugar, so you need less insulin to do the job. Unfortunately, levels of chromium in the body tend to decrease with age.

- Take 500 micrograms of chromium twice a day.

- **Take a multivitamin:** Studies show people with diabetes who take multivitamins decrease infections (specifically flu and intestinal and respiratory infections). In a study of more than 100 subjects over age 45, researchers found that only 17 of those taking the multivitamin developed an infection, while 93 percent of those taking the placebo became sick. The finding applied to both people with diabetes and those who are obese.[16]

- **Use magnesium:** Many people with diabetes have a deficiency in magnesium; supplements (even at low doses) tend to minimize complications related to the disease.
  - Take 300 milligrams of magnesium chloride daily.

Control Diabetes with Herbs

- **Gymnema sylvestre:** This herb can help to improve or control type 2 diabetes. In one study, 23 percent of the patients were able to discontinue their oral insulin and all the patients were able to reduce their insulin dosage. Researchers suggest that GS may regenerate or repair the pancreatic beta cells that produce insulin.[17]
  - Take 100 milligrams twice a day.

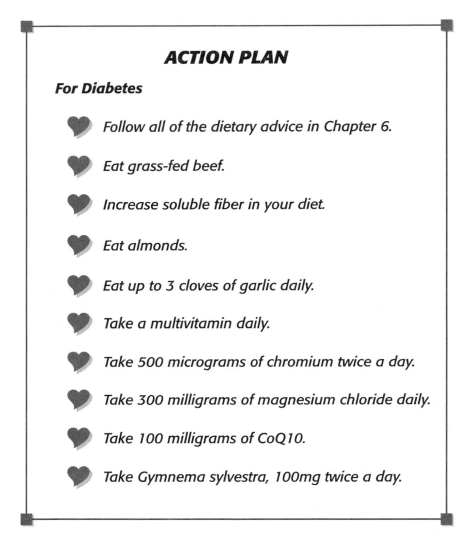

ACTION PLAN

For Diabetes

- Follow all of the dietary advice in Chapter 6.

- Eat grass-fed beef.

- Increase soluble fiber in your diet.

- Eat almonds.

- Eat up to 3 cloves of garlic daily.

- Take a multivitamin daily.

- Take 500 micrograms of chromium twice a day.

- Take 300 milligrams of magnesium chloride daily.

- Take 100 milligrams of CoQ10.

- Take Gymnema sylvestra, 100mg twice a day.

Diabetes often occurs because other health problems go unresolved, just as we see with heart disease. The rate of type 2 diabetes has tripled in the last 30 years. Much of this is due to the dramatic increase in obesity. Overweight people have a five-fold greater risk of diabetes.[18]

You will find a program for losing body fat later in this chapter. Many people with maturity-onset diabetes also have a chronic loss of muscle. Restoring muscle is critical to restoring your youthful metabolism.

Build Muscle

If you tested low in lean body mass in the tests in Chapter 5, you can increase the size of your muscles using resistance training. Since you can easily and gradually increase resistance, you can stimulate muscle growth.

If you've practiced standard weight-training programs in the past, you've probably trained your muscles to tense. While this may make you look good, it does nothing for your health. *The Doctor's Heart Cure's* muscle-building program helps you retrain your muscles to serve you in ways nature intended.

Build Muscle Mass

For you to be fit, it's important to develop and maintain muscle mass as well as cardiovascular capacity. Resistance exercise builds and preserves lean muscles. *The Doctor's Heart Cure's* specialized resistance training program in this chapter helps you reach your optimal state of muscular conditioning.

This plan differs from other muscle building programs in healthy and functional ways. When most people think of weight training, they think of gym exercises for the arms, chest, and shoulders. While these exercises can build some muscle, they are not a central part of this program. Why?

Because your upper body contains only about 15 percent of your body's total muscle mass. If you increased their size by 200 percent, you would not notice a measurable difference in your body's total muscle mass. To increase muscle mass in a meaningful way, work your large muscle groups.

Your largest muscles are your quadriceps, the muscles on the front of your thighs. The second largest are the gluteus muscles of your buttocks, and third are the hamstrings on the back of your thighs. All three of your biggest muscles flex and extend your hips. The key to building substantial muscle mass is to exercise these large muscles.

Use It or Lose It

The natural trend (if you don't do anything about it) is to lose muscle sarcopenia. While many people assume that their muscles will atrophy as they grow older, this doesn't have to be the case.

Without training, you lose muscle mass. Every decade from age forty on, the average person loses three pounds of muscle tissue. This gradual change in body composition from muscle to fat changes the shape of your body. It may not change your weight on the scales because muscle is denser than fat. Doing resistance exercises regularly helps you keep muscle mass and a more youthful figure. Otherwise, you go from firm to flabby, even if you weigh the same.

Training also staves off changes in body composition by raising the Basal Metabolic Rate (BMR), or the number of calories your body burns at rest. The more muscle you have, the higher your metabolic rate, the more calories you burn, and the easier it is to fight flab. At age twenty, the average woman has 23 percent body fat; the average man, 18 percent. At thirty-five, those fat figures jump to 30 and 25 percent, respectively. And by age sixty, the average woman is 44 percent fat and the average man, 38 percent fat.

To slow this shift from muscle to fat, do muscle building exercises. Important note: Studies show that even people who maintain their aerobic fitness still lose muscle mass – about one pound of muscle every two years after age twenty – if they don't diversify their workouts to include muscle building exercises.

Fortunately, it's never too late to build muscle. A recent study looked at the effects of exercise on sarcopenia in the elderly. Twenty-one frail, elderly participants took part in a resistance-training program for 11 weeks. After the program, their muscle mass increased by up to 60 percent. In addition, they demonstrated an overall improvement in balance, strength, and physical ability, making them less likely to fall.[19]

In fact, regular muscle training virtually stops the aging process when it comes to your muscles. For example, one study found that seventy-year-old men who trained since middle age had as much muscle on average, as twenty-year-old men who didn't do muscle training exercise. The more shrinkage of muscle you have, the greater your results will be. Frail octogenarians can double their muscle mass in just a couple of months.

Training Tips

- **Start with a training weight of about 70 to 80 percent of the maximum weight that you can lift.** If the heaviest weight you can lift in a certain maneuver is twenty-five pounds, your training weight for that exercise is fifteen to twenty pounds. Lift that weight eight to twelve times. Once you can lift a weight twenty times, move up to a heavier weight.

This approach helps build "fast twitch" or "white" muscle fibers, which are responsible for strength. Muscles also contain "slow twitch" or "red" muscle fibers, which help with exercise endurance. To build these muscles, include weight sets that are lighter and perform more repetitions. For this approach, do your initial weight set at 70 to 80 percent of your maximum, then mix in a set that is 40 to 60 percent of maximum (or lower). It is natural to feel achy a day or two after working a muscle group in this way. If your muscles feel painful longer than that, talk to a physical trainer or another health professional for advice.

- **Do multiple drop sets.** One set of each exercise is almost as effective as multiple sets in building muscle and boosting metabolism. However, to build muscle faster, follow a high-intensity strategy: After finishing the set, reduce the weight by ten pounds and do three or four more. Continue these drop sets by lowering the weight with each set for 3 or 4 sets with only a minute or less of rest between sets. A two-month study found that people who followed the high-intensity strategy were able to lift 25 pounds more than they could before. People who used the one-set approach were able to lift just 15 pounds more.

- **Work your largest muscle groups first.** Start with your legs and back and then exercise your hips and calves.

- **Alternate upper and lower body workouts.** Three workouts per week is the basic recommendation for building muscle. However, many people find it easiest to do a split routine, alternating between working the muscles in the upper body one day and the lower body the next.

- **Take it slow and easy.** Take about six seconds for each repetition of an exercise: two seconds for the first half of the maneuver and four for the return to the original position.

- **Use good form.** Doing an exercise ineffectively can cause muscle damage and injury.

- **Breathe!** Don't hold your breath. Holding your breath can cause a dangerous rise in blood pressure, then a sudden drop when you release your breath, possibly causing light-headedness or fainting. Inhale and then exhale during the exertion phase of the movement and inhale during the release.

- **Start comfortably.** If you are wary of free weights, start with weight-lifting machines. You can use dumb-bells for a variety of exercises. Working with a personal trainer can help you establish good form.

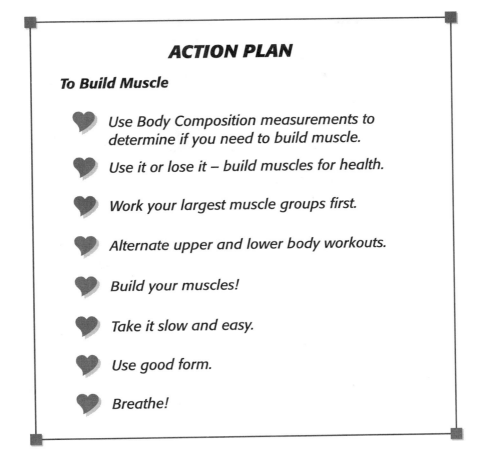

ACTION PLAN

To Build Muscle

Use Body Composition measurements to determine if you need to build muscle.

Use it or lose it – build muscles for health.

Work your largest muscle groups first.

Alternate upper and lower body workouts.

Build your muscles!

Take it slow and easy.

Use good form.

Breathe!

Lose Weight Naturally

Carrying extra body fat puts you at greater risk of a number of health problems, including heart disease, diabetes, high blood pressure, stroke, gallbladder disease, hemorrhoids, varicose veins, and kidney and liver problems.

More than half of all Americans are overweight and 50 million of those are obese, despite obsessing about what they put in their mouths. As any veteran of the battle of the bulge knows, obesity can be very difficult to control using traditional approaches to diet.

To lose weight naturally and pleasantly, begin by follow the eating plan described in Chapter 6 then add the tips you find in this chapter. They have worked with thousands of patients. You can make them work for you, too, more easily than you may imagine. Don't assume that to lose weight you have to deny yourself food. This approach may lead to short-term results, but it eventually backfires. Make easy lifestyle changes that you can sustain and they will serve you well for the rest of your life.

A Surprising Secret Which Makes Weight Loss Healthier and Easier

If you want to lose fat and keep it off, don't bother counting calories. This patient's story illustrates how obsessing over calories won't make you lean. This is a lesson that took me a while to learn.

About 15 years ago, a young woman came to the Center for Health and Wellness wanting to lose weight. She said, "You helped two of my friends lose a lot of weight, but it doesn't work for me. No matter how little I eat, my weight just keeps going up. I'm only 5'2" and I weigh 170. That's the most I've ever weighed, and I've been dieting." She worked 10 hours a day as a waitress and worked out for 90 minutes five times a week.

She restricted her diet to 1,600 calories per day, wrote down everything she ate and came back in two weeks. When she returned, she showed a detailed record of her progress, including her weight gain of two pounds.

She cut her intake to 1,400 calories per day and came back in two weeks. Once again, she followed the program – and gained two more pounds.

Next, she slashed her calories to 1,200 – and then to a mere 1,000 per day – but she continued to gain weight. In addition, she lacked energy, stopped working out, and felt more depressed than she did before she came.

Ultimately, she quit the program. She never came back and she never returned calls from the Center for Health and Wellness. This story is an extreme example that starving yourself thin is a losing strategy. Your body will fight you, and in the end, it will win; this is why conventional diets don't work. Five out of six people who try to lose weight fail. Of those who do lose weight, more than 90 percent gain all the weight back within two years.

If you go hungry to force your body to lose weight, your body fights you every step of the way. The body responds to starvation by doing everything it can to preserve your fat. If you have the strength of will to stick to this starvation plan and lose weight, you also lose important muscle, bone, and even vital organ mass.

To lose weight and get healthier in the process, reset your body's natural weight regulator. You can understand the mechanisms your body uses to set your weight. By changing your diet and exercise routines, you can provide a new set of signals for your body to establish your optimal weight naturally. You don't have to eat less, just eat differently.

Experience with another patient underscores the different way that foods affect weight gain. This man also weighed 170 pounds, and he desperately wanted to gain weight. Experts told him to eat more protein to put on more muscle. He said he kept adding protein to his plate, but he couldn't gain an ounce. His food log was astounding. He ate a dozen egg whites and 24 ounces of steak every day! He drank a 40-ounce protein shake twice a day, and between meals he gobbled pure-protein snacks and as much as 36 ounces of canned tuna! When his calories were added up, he ate over 5,000 calories a day for the 12 weeks on his record yet still managed to lose six pounds.

He wasn't burning off the calories in the gym, either. He worked out with weights three times a week for thirty to forty minutes. He avoided cardio exercise because he didn't want to burn the calories.

Could these two patients – one who couldn't lose weight and one who couldn't gain – have differed very dramatically in their Basal Metabolic Rate (BMR), or the rate they burn calories at rest? Research shows only marginal variations in BMR, nothing nearly wide enough to account for these dramatic differences.

The answer – and the key to effective weight loss – is this: *To make weight loss easy and healthy*, eat more protein than your body needs. Eating more protein than the body needs tells your body that you have plenty to eat – you are NOT starving – and you do not need to store fat. Instead, your body can burn fat stores for other purposes.

What these two patients experienced has repeated with thousands of additional patients at the Center for Health and Wellness. To lose weight, eat more than your daily requirement for protein. (For a complete set of dietary recommendations, see Chapter 6.)

How Much Protein Is Enough?

If your weight is good where it is, eat about a half gram of protein per pound of bodyweight. If you want to lose weight, increase your protein consumption to one gram per pound of desired bodyweight. For example, if you weigh 180 pounds, eat 180 grams of protein per day. Once you achieve the weight-loss you want, decrease your protein to about a half-gram per pound.

To all the nutritionists who want to say that this is more protein that a person needs – that's the point. To lose weight, eat more protein than your body needs.

Choose lean sources of protein such as steak, turkey, chicken, and fish. Choose carbohydrates wisely, as we talked about in Chapter 6.

Eat Good Carbs Only

You have seen that cutting calories is not the best way to lose weight. And that eating enough protein can "throw a switch" that will get your body to burn the fat it stores.

Now let's look at the last piece of the fat-loss puzzle. By eating the "right" kinds of carbs you can induce your body to make and store less fat. This is a tremendous fat-blasting secret few people know about.

Understand How the Glycemic Index Affects Your Weight

The Glycemic Index ranks foods on how rapidly they spike your blood sugar levels. The index is expressed in percentage terms. A food with a glycemic index of 50 percent causes half of the rapid rise in blood sugar that glucose (pure natural sugar) does.

Why don't you want to spike your blood sugar levels? Because when you do, your body starts converting the food you eat into fat. The higher the glycemic index of the food you eat, the more fat you'll make from it even if it has an equal number of calories. Even if they have heard of the glycemic index, most of the patients I treat think sweets are the trouble. This is incorrect.

The real problem is with starches. They not only produce more blood sugar but they cause a much more prolonged elevation of sugar and insulin than simple sugars do. Look again at the glycemic index in Chapter 6. If you have a tendency toward high insulin, body fat or diabetes it is even more important to use your food as your medicine.

THE FDA AND SUPPLEMENT LABELS

In 1994, Congress passed the Dietary Supplement Health and Education Act (DSHEA). The law allows manufacturers to bring naturally occurring supplements to market without prior Food and Drug Administration (FDA) approval as long as they don't make health claims. It has succeeded in allowing a rapid expansion in new, natural supplements. But with the responsibility of determining the safety and claims of a product in the manufacturers' hands, it's "buyer beware."

Since there are no strict guidelines for managing supplements, you need to know how to separate decent manufacturers from shady ones. Good companies are willing to share research on their product ingredients. Many manufactures get their products lab tested by independent sources and will make the testing results available to you.

Lose Fat Now and Live Longer

You'll get around to losing those extra pounds... tomorrow. Right? Well, consider that being overweight in middle age equates to a shorter life expectancy. According to a study published in the January 2003 issue of the *Annals of Internal Medicine*, Dutch researchers analyzed data taken from 3,457 subjects from 1948 to 1990. Obese middle-aged men lived an average of 5.8 years less than slimmer men did. Regardless of whether the men were slim in their youth, if they were overweight in the 30s and 40s, they lost years off their life.[20]

Five Simple Weight-Loss Tips

These simple changes can help you lose weight – and keep it off.

- Eat breakfast every day. Not eating breakfast increases your risk of becoming obese by a stunning 450 percent.
- Snack in the afternoon. Eating at least one midday snack slashes your risk of obesity by 39 percent.
- Drink water with every meal. Each time you sit down to a meal, put a full glass of water by your plate. As you hunger is satisfied, you will feel thirsty.
- Don't snack in front of the TV. This bad habit distracts you for your food and encourages mindless overeating.
- Plan your meals. You will make healthier food choices if you think ahead and plan you meals. Eating should be a pleasure.

A slender, fit body is not reserved for the young. Stay lean and healthy throughout your entire life – starting today.

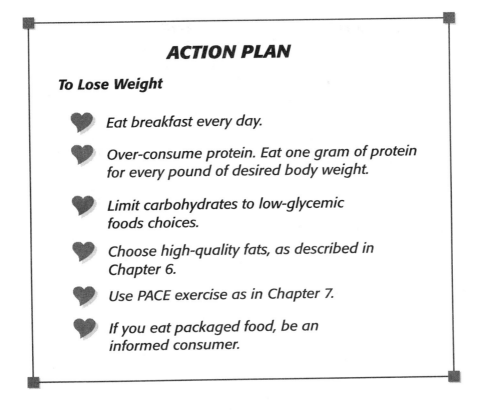

ACTION PLAN

To Lose Weight

💜 *Eat breakfast every day.*

💜 *Over-consume protein. Eat one gram of protein for every pound of desired body weight.*

💜 *Limit carbohydrates to low-glycemic foods choices.*

💜 *Choose high-quality fats, as described in Chapter 6.*

💜 *Use PACE exercise as in Chapter 7.*

💜 *If you eat packaged food, be an informed consumer.*

Footnotes Chapter 11

1 Auer W, Eiber A, Hostkorn E, et al. Hypertension and hyperlipidaemia: Garlic helps in mild cases. *British Journal of Clinical Practical Supplements.* 1990 Aug; 69:3-6.

2 Kurl S, et al. Plasma Vitamin C modifies the association between hypertension and risk of stroke. *Journal of the American Medical Association.* 2002 Sep 18; 288(11):1333.

3 Associated Press, Vitamin C Can Lower Blood Pressure, December 21, 1999. www.intellihealth.com/IH

4 Walker AF, Marakis G, Morris AP, and Robinson PA. Promising hypotensive effect of hawthorn extract: A randomized double-blind pilot study of mild, essential hypertension. *Phytotherapy Research.* 2002 Jan; 16(1):48-54.

5 Blekas G, Vassilakis C, Harizanis C, et al. Biophenols in table olives. *Journal of Agriculture and Food Chemistry.* 2002 Jun 19; 50(13):3588-3692.

6 Jenkins DJ, Kendall CW, Marchie A, et al. Effects of a dietary portfolio of cholesterol-lowering foods vs. Lovastatin on serum lipids and C-reactive protein. *Journal of the American Medical Association.* 2003 Jul; 290(4):502-510.

7 Waladkhani AR and Clemens MR. Effect of dietary phytochemicals on cancer development (review). *International Journal of Molecular Medicine.* 1998 Apr; 1(4):747-753.

8 Vega-Lopez S, Vidal-Quintanar RL and Fernandez ML. Sex and hormonal status influence plasma lipid responses to psyllium. *American Journal of Clinical Nutrition.* 2001 Oct; 74(4):435-441.

9 Rogers S, et al. Triglyceride lowering effect of MaxEPA fish lipid concentrate: a multicentre, placebo-controlled, double-blind study. *Clinical Chimera Acta.* 1988 Dec 30; 178:251-259.

10 Furman B, Rosenblat M, Hayek T, et al. Ginger extract consumption reduces plasma cholesterol, inhibits LDL oxidation and attenuates development of atherosclerosis in atherosclerotic apolipoprotein E-deficient mice. *Journal of Nutrition.* 2000 May; 130(5):1124-1131.

11 Urizar NL and Moore DD. Gugulipid: a natural cholesterol-lowering agent. *Annual Review of Nutrition.* 2003; 23:303-313.

12 French P, et al. Fatty acid composition, including conjugated linoleic acid, of intramuscular fat from steers offered grazed grass, grass silage, or concentrate-based diets. *Journal of Animal Science.* 2000; 78:2849-2855

13 Dhiman T, et al. Conjugated linoleic acid from cows fed different diets. *Journal of Dairy Science.* 1999; 82(10):2146-2156

14 Smith G. Dietary supplementation of Vitamin E to cattle to improve shelf life and case life of beef for domestic and international markets. Colorado State University

15 Wein MA, Sabate JM, Ikle DN, et al. Almonds vs complex carbohydrates in a weight reduction program. International *Journal of Obesity and Related Metabolic Disorders.* 2003 Mar; 28(3) 1365-1372.

16 Barringer TA, Kirk JK, Santaniello AC, et al. Effect of a multivitamin and mineral supplement on infection and quality of life. A randomized, double-blind, placebo-controlled trial. *Annals of Internal Medicine.* 2003 Mar 4; 138(5): 365-371.

17 Baskaran K, Kizar Ahamath B, et al. Antidiabetic effect of a leaf extract from Gymnema slvestre in non-insulin-dependent diabetes mellitus patients. *Journal of Ethnopharmacology.* 1990 Oct; 30(3):295-300.

18 National Institute of Diabetes & Digestive & Kidney Disease, Diet and Exercise Dramatically Delay Type 2 Diabetes: Diabetes Medication Metformin Also Effective, http://www.niddk.nih.gov/welcome/releases/8_8_01.htm

19 LaStoya PC, Ewy GA. Pierotti DD, et al. The positive effects of negative work: increased muscle strength and decreased fall risk in a frail elderly population. *Journal of Gerontology and Biological Science And Medical Science.* 2003 May; 58(5):M417-418.

20 Peeters A, Barendregt JJ, Willekins F, et al. Obesity in adulthood and its consequences for life expectancy: a life-table analysis. *Annals of Internal Medicine.* 2003 Jan 7; 138(1):24-32.

12

Heart Health Now: An 8 Week Program

Thousands of patients have reversed their heart disease, regained their vitality, and changed their lives. You can build heart health, too. *The Doctor's Heart Cure* Plan is easy to follow. You can eat foods you love, meet your exercise goal in 10 to 15 minutes a day, and take a few safe and health-enhancing supplements once or twice a day.

A special note: Don't let an inherited genetic predisposition to heart problems discourage you – use it to your advantage. Take action now to prevent and reverse heart disease, despite any inherited vulnerability. My experience gives me faith that your genetic inheritance need not dictate your future health. Recently a study published in the July 2003 issue of *The American College of Cardiology* proves that for heart disease, genetics is not destiny. Researchers analyzed 684 identical twins and found that the twin who exercised regularly had a significantly lower risk of developing heart disease than the twin who did not exercise, despite having the same genetics.

Let's think about this for a minute. In this study, the twins didn't follow the most effective exercise program for cardiovascular conditioning. They did not change their eating habits or take nutritional supplements. They had no testing of oxidation or inflammation. Yet if one single intervention like exercise can make such a difference in genetically identical individuals, just imagine what a difference your comprehensive *Doctor's Heart Cure* Plan can make.

Your genetic predisposition may be the hand you were dealt, but through your choices, you decide which cards to play. Your ultimate success depends not on who you are, but on what you do.

Take Action Today

- Plan your eating and exercise activities one day ahead.
- Center your plans around foods you enjoy and exercise that brings you pleasure.
- Start the day right with brief cardio exercise before breakfast.
- Eat a high-protein breakfast.
- Train for strength and muscle mass either before lunch or before dinner.
- Make a portion of your physical activity recreation every day.
- Plan dinner around high-quality protein (steak, roast, fish, or chicken).
- Take time to enjoy your family and friends.
- Every evening take time to reflect on today's progress and plan tomorrow's accomplishments.

Start by crediting the good features of your health to your daily habits. Then commit to building, reinforcing and strengthening those features with better habits. Like everyone else, you will slip up sometimes, miss workouts and make poor food choices. Don't expect every day to be a universal success, but plan each day as if it will be. Forgive yourself for periodic indiscretions and then get back on track the next day. Optimal health is a journey, not a destination. So remember ... enjoy the ride.

Your Doctor's Heart Cure Plan

Here's a week-by-week checklist for putting your plan into action. To review specific information on each of these action steps, see the corresponding chapters.

Week 1

Assess Where You Are:
- Measure your body composition: Set a goal of no more than 25 percent body fat. Following this program will help you attain and maintain this goal.
- Get the following tests done by your doctor annually:
    - Homocysteine levels: Aim for less than 8 mmol per liter.
    - C-reactive protein: Aim for below 1 unit; lower is better.
    - CoQ10: Aim for 2.5 to 3.5 nanograms per milliliter. You will probably have to supplement with CoQ10 to reach this goal.
    - Insulin: Aim for 10 micro units per milliliter or less.

Choose Healthy Foods:
- Eat quality protein.
    - Eat protein at every meal.
    - Choose free-farmed meat and poultry.
    - Eat seafood, especially Alaskan or wild salmon.
    - Eat eggs.
    - Drink organic milk.

Exercise for your Heart: PACE™ – Four times weekly
- Exercise 20 minutes.
    - Exercise 20 minutes at intensity level 2

Give your Heart Nutrients
- CoQ10: Take 100 milligrams daily if you have heart disease.

Week 2

Begin to Get the Feel of Varying PACE™: Four times a week
- Exercise 20 minutes.
    - Exercise 20 minutes: experiment with increasing and decreasing intensity levels.

Add a Multivitamin:
- Continue to take CoQ10.
- Multi-vitamin: Take a complete multi-vitamin/mineral supplement daily.

Week 3

Begin to Decrease Insulin Stimulating Carbohydrates
- Continue to eat plenty of protein from Week 1.
- Choose quality carbohydrate.
  - Eat low-glycemic foods. All real vegetables and berries are okay. NOTE: Potatoes (a tuber) and corn (a grain) are not vegetables.
  - Avoid all high-glycemic foods. Do not eat grain products (cereals and breads).

Begin Using Interval Exercise: PACE™ – Four times a week
- Exercise 20 minutes:
  - Exercise 8 minutes at intensity level 3
  - Rest 4 minutes at intensity level 2
  - Exercise 8 minutes at intensity level 4

Add Energy Nutrient:
- Continue with CoQ10 and multivitamin.
- Add L-Carnitine for more energy: Take 500 milligrams daily.

Week 4

- Continue to eat excess protein and low glycemic vegetables and berries.

Begin to Gradually Increase the PACE™: Four times a week
- Exercise 20 minutes:
  - Exercise 8 minutes at intensity level 4

- Rest for 4 minutes at intensity level 2
- Exercise for 8 minutes at intensity level 5

Add Heart Nutrients:
- Continue with CoQ10, multi-vitamins and L-Carnitine.
- Add L-Arginine: 500 milligrams daily.

Week 5

Begin to Improve the Quality of Dietary Fat:
- Continue to eat excess protein and limit carbs.
- Begin to choose highest quality fat.
  - Increase Omega-3 fats. Good sources of Omega-3s include grass fed meat, free-range poultry, wild fish, olives, eggs, nuts, and avocadoes. NOTE: Peanuts are not true nuts.
  - Decrease Omega-6 fats (grain-fed and processed meats).
  - Avoid *trans* fats (margarine, processed vegetable oils, pre-packaged baked goods).

Begin Shortening your PACE™ Intervals: Four times weekly
- Exercise 18 minutes:
  - Exercise 6 minutes at intensity level 4
  - Rest 2 minutes at intensity level 2
  - Exercise 4 minutes at intensity level 5
  - Rest 2 minutes at intensity level 2
  - Exercise 4 minutes at intensity level 4

Begin Strengthening with bodyweight Movements: 4 times a week
- Monday and Thursday: Lower Body
  - Alternating lunges
  - Squats
  - Squat leaps
  - Leg levers
  - Back flutter kicks
  - Scissors

- Tuesday and Friday: Upper Body
  - Push-ups
  - Arm haulers
  - Pull-ups
  - Dips
  - Crunches

Supplements:
- Continue to take CoQ10, multi-vitamin/mineral supplement, L-Carnitine, and L-Arginine.
- Tocopherols and tocotrienols: Take 400 IU of vitamin E with at least 5 milligrams of mixed tocopherols and tocotrienols daily.

Week 6

Diet:
- Continue to eat excess protein, limit carbs and eat quality fats.

Balance exercise and rest intervals: PACE™ – Four times weekly
- Exercise 20 minutes:
  - Exercise 4 minutes at intensity level 4
  - Rest 4 minutes at intensity level 2
  - Exercise 4 minutes at intensity level 5
  - Rest 4 minutes at intensity level 2
  - Exercise 4 minutes at intensity level 4

Keep strengthening with bodyweight Exercises – 4 times a week
- Monday and Thursday: Legs and Lower Body
  - Follow suggestions in Week 5
- Tuesday and Friday: Upper Body and Core
  - Follow suggestions in Week 5

Supplements:
- Continue to take CoQ10, complete multi-vitamin/mineral supplement, L-Carnitine, L-Arginine, and 400 IU of vitamin E with at least 5 milligrams of mixed tocopherols and tocotrienols daily.
  - Vitamin C: Take 500 milligrams twice daily with food.

Week 7

Diet:
- Continue to eat good protein, limit your carbs and use high quality fats.
- Avoid problems created by the modern food industry.
  - Avoid genetically modified foods.
  - Avoid all "low-fat" packaged foods.
  - Do not overcook your food.

Shorten exercise and rest periods: PACE™ – Four times weekly
- Exercise 20 minutes:
  - Exercise 4 minutes at intensity level 4
  - Rest 3 minutes at intensity level 2
  - Exercise 3 minutes at intensity level 5
  - Rest 3 minutes at intensity level 2
  - Exercise 2 minutes at intensity level 6
  - Rest 2 minutes at intensity level 2
  - Exercise 3 minutes at intensity level 5

- **Continue to use bodyweight Exercises** – 4 times a week
- Monday and Thursday: Legs and Lower Body
  - Follow suggestions in Week 5
- Tuesday and Friday: Upper Body and Core
  - Follow suggestions in Week 5

Supplements:
- Continue to take CoQ10, a complete multi-vitamin/mineral supplement, L-Carnitine, L-Arginine, Vitamin E with mixed tocopherols and tocotrienols, and Vitamin C.

Week 8

Diet:
- Make your on-going diet one of good protein, limited carbs, and high quality fats. Avoid food industry products which cause problems.

Exercise: Maintain exercise schedule for PACE™ – Four times weekly
- Exercise 20 minutes:
  - Exercise 4 minutes at intensity level 4
  - Rest 3 minutes at intensity level 2
  - Exercise 3 minutes at intensity level 5
  - Rest 3 minutes at intensity level 2
  - Exercise 2 minutes at intensity level 6
  - Rest 2 minutes at intensity level 2
  - Exercise 3 minutes at intensity level 5

bodyweight Exercises – 4 times a week
- Monday and Thursday: Legs and Lower Body
  - Follow suggestions in Week 5
- Tuesday and Friday: Upper Body and Core
  - Follow suggestions in Week 5

Supplements:
- On a daily basis take: CoQ10, a complete multi-vitamin/mineral supplement, L-Carnitine, L-Arginine, Vitamin E with mixed tocopherols and tocotrienols, and Vitamin C.

Design Your Own Plan

Decide on some favorite physical exercises and then create your program. The different patterns of exercises you can do are countless. Split up your exercise by major muscle groups.

For cardiopulmonary capacity, remember to include your PACE™ program in your regimen. For building muscle, use resistance training, focusing on the big muscles of the back and legs. That's where muscle bulk has the most benefits. Build your functional strength using your own bodyweight. Calisthenics are the most effective and safest way to do this. You can find descriptions of PACE™ programs and bodyweight calisthenics in Chapter 7. To build muscle, add the exercise plan in Chapter 11.

My Favorite Grand Workout Plan

Day 1	Resistance Train Legs and Back
Day 2	Calisthenics
Day 3	PACE
Day 4	Resistance Train Back and Legs
Day 5	Calisthenics
Day 6	PACE
Day 7	Rest

The Doctor's Heart Cure is a lifelong plan that helps you live a longer and healthier life. Realistically, you will only follow this plan when you can incorporate it into your life easily and enjoyably. This plan works in the long run because it is an enjoyable and sustainable *way of life*. It is, after all, only recreating the diet and physical practices of our ancestors. You feel fulfilled rather than deprived, energized rather than fatigued, and mended rather than medicated.

DEAR DIARY: BUILD HEART HEALTH!

6:30 a.m.: Wake up early and get moving.
Ben Franklin was right; rising with the sun is profoundly health-enhancing. I wake up when my alarm sounds at 6:30 a.m. I'm just as tempted to hit the snooze button and doze off as anyone else. I plan

ahead by putting my running shoes and exercise log next to the bed at night. When I wake up, I see them and they remind me to go for my goals. After I climb out of bed, I check my e-mail while indulging in a quick cup of coffee. By 7 a.m. I'm out the door and off to the gym.

7:15 a.m.: Keep in mind that quality is more important than quantity when exercising.

As part of my PACE™ program for heart health, I challenge myself physically a little more each day to build larger lung and heart capacity. I vary my workout to avoid boredom and overuse injuries, and today I plan to bicycle. I start with a 2-minute warm up at a gentle pace, then accelerate to a moderate pace (an intensity of 5 on a 10-point scale) for 1 minute. Next, I recover for 1 minute by working at an easy pace (an intensity of 3 on a 10-point scale). I repeat this alternating cycle of high- and moderate-intensity several more times, gradually increasing the intensity of my effort during the high-intensity portions of the workout. Throughout my workout, I remind myself to breathe deeply. Today, I am going for a 10. I pedal as hard as I can for 30 seconds. I feel an intense burn in the front of my thighs as the lactic acid builds up in my quadriceps. This is what I want; I can feel this improving the oxygen-delivering capacity of my heart and lungs. My total workout time: 12 minutes.

7:45 a.m.: Nothing can take the place of a high-protein breakfast.

For breakfast, I enjoy a 3-egg omelet with salmon and a glass of water. I take 10 grams of glutamine to prevent muscle breakdown and boost growth hormone. I also take 1,000 milligrams of vitamin C and a combination multi-vitamin, multi-mineral, multi-antioxidant supplement with my breakfast.

12:30 p.m.: Enjoy extra protein at lunch.

During my lunch break, I stop by a local restaurant and place an order for a seafood salad with extra tuna. (Since I'm working the big muscles of my legs today, I want extra protein after my workout.)

3:00 p.m.: Snack for energy in the afternoon.

After working a couple more hours, I take an afternoon break. I take a deep breath and snack on a couple of ounces of Longhorn cheese, one of my favorites. I finish my workday, have a brief meeting and head for home.

7:00 p.m.: Time to dine: Don't be afraid of red meat.

I dine with family and friends who know I eat grass-fed red meat or wild game almost every day. (Remember, 70 - 85 percent of the calories in our ancestor's diet came from red meat.) We end the meal with a bowl of ice cream and sliced peaches, topped with whipped cream and walnuts. I'm not concerned about the fat, but I do try to choose a low-glycemic fruit. (Peaches have a glycemic index less than half of that of whole wheat bread.) I also buy ice cream without added sugar.

9:00 p.m.: Close the day with a period of quiet reflection.

When I can, I end my day with a contemplative walk around my neighborhood for relaxation. Psychoanalyst Sigmund Freud claimed that people need three things to be happy: relationships, occupations, and recreations – or love, work, and play. Today, many people focus too much energy on work, neglecting love and play. To live a balanced life, make time for all three of these essential ingredients of happiness. Plan your health and fitness goals with the same spirit you plan recreation. If possible, involve family and friends.

11:00 p.m.: Rest for your health.

By 11 p.m., I'm ready to hit the sack. I take a few minutes to think about what I'd like to accomplish tomorrow, what I want to eat, and how I want to exercise. I write down my achievements for the day, and I set tomorrow's goals in my daily log. I reflect for a few minutes about my day, then clear my mind and drift off to sleep.

Keep a log of your daily progress.

Whether working with athletes as a strength coach, personal trainer, consultant, or as an integrative medical doctor, there is no better predictor of long-term success of reaching health goals (or any other goals for that matter), than whether or not someone is willing to keep a daily log. To succeed, write down your goals. Use a log book to keep track of your daily progress.

When you write your goals, you make a commitment to yourself to work toward those goals. When you record your progress, you acknowledge your achievements and recognize you are taking the steps necessary to transform yourself and become the healthy person you want to be.

You can use the same log for planning and recording your results. Do your planning in pencil, then write over the words in pen when you do what is written. You can use a section of a daily planner or keep a separate fitness journal.

Start Now and Make Today the Best Day of Your Life

There is an ancient Chinese proverb: Knowing and not doing is the same as not knowing. You have your plan. You know what to do. Now is the time to act.

This system will make heart-healthy habits automatic. The tips that follow are self-coaching tools. They give you a specific plan of action to reach your goals effortlessly and regularly. They help you get started. Then you can go on to come up with some of your own as well.

Plan your exercise and eating for the following day.

Important accomplishments start with planning. Take five minutes at the end of every day to plan your exercises and meals for the next day. Now, you won't always stick to the plan perfectly. But if you fail to plan, you will tend to skip workouts and munch on whatever food you can find at the moment. Consider your plan as a self-coaching tool. Don't feel guilty when the plan changes. Setting reasonable daily goals helps provide direction for your day.

Before going to bed, plan and write down in a daily planner your exercise for the next day. Do it like you would schedule a business meeting. Now look at your plan for the day. See if you have to make any adjustments to be sure to get your exercise on the schedule accomplished. For example, you may note a long day at the office and decide to plan 10 minutes of PACE™ in the morning before going to work and a brief strength-training workout at lunch.

Also plan your meals for the day. For breakfast, you might plan to have scrambled eggs with leftover salmon from tonight's dinner. For lunch, you might plan to pick up a seafood salad 'to go' from the restaurant near your work. You plan to have steak for dinner so you make a note to pull them from the freezer and start the marinade.

By planning, you make conscious decisions about reaching you goals, rather than reacting to the moment which can allow circumstances to dictate your choices.

Now you have a plan. You hold the keys to a healthy life and heart the natural way. Take action now. Take a step toward a more robust heart, lungs and blood vessels today and every day.

Let us hear how you use this book to boost your health or that of a loved one. Mail to DrSearsResearch@AOL.com. You may see your own success recorded in future publications, and help others achieve their own *Doctor's Heart Cure*. May you play hard, live long and go far!

APPENDIX A

A Primer on
Heart Disease

Y our heart and circulatory system feed every cell in your body with
life-giving oxygen. This complex 12,400-mile network of arteries,
veins, and blood vessels circulates blood from your heart to the farthest
reaches of your body. In a healthy adult, the heart beats about 100,000
times a day, pumping the equivalent of more than 4,000 gallons of blood.
That's an impressive accomplishment – one that underscores the importance
of maintaining a well-tuned heart and circulatory system.

But all too often the system fails. Heart attacks, atherosclerosis, congestive heart failure, strokes, and other circulatory disease claim about one
million lives a year. In addition, a huge number of Americans – more than
63 million – live with some form of heart or blood vessel disease. Heart disease kills more people than any other ailment.

Although the risk of heart attack and cardiovascular disease increases
with age, about a fifth of the deaths occur among people under age 65.
Fortunately, many of these deaths can be prevented by lifestyle changes,
and by avoiding or minimizing the factors that increase the risk of cardiovascular disease.

Heart Attack

The heart is a muscle, and like any other muscle, it needs oxygen to stay
alive. When all or part of the heart muscle dies due to lack of oxygen, it is
called a heart attack, or *myocardial infarction.*

Blood clots cause many heart attacks. When blood flows through an artery that has been narrowed by atherosclerosis, it slows down and tends to clot. When the clot becomes big enough, it cuts off the blood supply to the portion of the heart muscle below the clot, and that part of the heart muscle begins to die.

Heart attacks can also occur when the heartbeat becomes irregular. In severe cases this condition, known as arrhythmia, can prevent sufficient blood from reaching the heart muscle.

Angina

The pain starts with constriction in the center of the chest, then radiates to the throat, back, neck, jaw, and down the left arm. You break into a sweat, struggle for breath, and feel nauseated and dizzy. You may assume you're in the throes of The Big One – a full-blown, chest-crushing heart attack – but within ten minutes or so, it's over, and the pain gradually subsides. What you've experienced is not a heart attack but a full-blown attack or *angina pectoris*.

Some three million Americans suffer from angina, a painful episode that occurs when the heart muscle does not get enough oxygen. (This is known as *myocardial ischemia*.) Most angina attacks occur when the heart, damaged by high blood pressure and coronary artery disease, is stressed by physical exertion, emotional upset, excessive excitement, or even digestion of a heavy meal. Walking outside on a cold day, jogging to catch a bus, or experiencing particularly distressing news can trigger attacks. Angina attacks often serve as painful reminders that the heart has been damaged, and a full-blown heart attack may follow unless steps are taken to mend your ailing heart.

Atherosclerosis

"Hardening of the arteries," or atherosclerosis, involves the gradual buildup of fatty deposits or plaque in the arteries. The deposits narrow the arteries, reducing the blood supply to the heart and increasing the likelihood that a blood clot clogs up an arterial pathway and causes a heart attack.

Atherosclerosis is a three-step process. First, the arteries develop tiny tears due to the powerful contractions of the heart, especially in someone who has high blood pressure. Next, cholesterol in the blood sticks to the tears, slowly hardening into plaque, causing the arteries to become less flexible. Finally, these deposits narrow the arterial passages, reducing the blood supply to the heart muscle and other parts of the body.

The heart muscle is so efficient at extracting oxygen from the blood that many people develop severe coronary disease before any symptoms appear. In fact, the vessels can be 70 to 90 percent blocked before any symptoms occur, and often a heart attack is the first warning sign that something is wrong.

When it involves the coronary arteries, atherosclerosis causes heart attack. When it blocks blood flow to the brain, atherosclerosis causes stroke. And when it affects the arteries of the legs, it cause peripheral vascular disease.

Congestive Heart Failure

When the heart has been damaged and can no longer pump efficiently but has not failed outright, a person is suffering from congestive heart failure. When this occurs, the kidneys respond to the reduced blood circulation by retaining salt and water in the body, which adds additional stress to the heart and makes matters worse.

Congestive heart failure can affect either the right or left side of the heart. The left side pumps oxygen-rich blood from the lungs to the rest of the body. The right side of the heart pumps oxygen-depleted blood back from the body to the lungs that replenish the oxygen. When the left side of the heart is damaged, the blood backs up in the lungs, causing wheezing and shortness of breath (even during rest), fatigue, sleep disturbances, and a dry, hacking, nonproductive cough when lying down. When the right side of the heart is damaged, the blood collects in the legs and liver, causing swollen feet and ankles, swollen neck veins, pain below the ribs, fatigue, and lethargy.

Stroke

A stroke is like a heart attack in the brain. Just as a part of the heart dies when deprived of oxygen during a heart attack, so a part of the brain dies when deprived of oxygen during a stroke. A *thrombotic stroke* occurs when an artery in the brain is blocked by a clot or atherosclerosis; an *embolic stroke* occurs when a small clot (known as an embolus) forms elsewhere in the body and moves to the brain, where it lodges in an artery and blocks the flow of blood. A *hemorrhagic stroke* occurs when an artery ruptures, usually due to high blood pressure. While hemorrhagic strokes are less common – only about 20 percent of all strokes – they are much more lethal, causing about 50 percent of all stroke-related deaths.

In the aftermath of a stroke, the person loses the bodily function associated with the part of the brain the stroke destroyed. Symptoms of a stroke include slurred speech or loss of speech; sudden severe headache; double vision or blindness; sudden weakness or loss of sensation in the limbs; or loss of consciousness. The symptoms can occur over a period of a few minutes or hours, and they can occur on one side of the body or both.

Stroke is the nation's third leading cause of death and the leading cause of adult disability. Experts estimate that as many as 80 percent of all strokes can be prevented.

Recognizing the Warning Signs

Some people learn they have heart disease when they experience the chest-crushing pain of angina. But many others don't receive any warning – until they have their first heart attack.

Heart attack victims often delay seeking medical help, frequently with fatal results. The cells of your heart require a constant supply of blood. If they don't get it, the cells die. The number of cells that die during a heart attack determines if you live or die. If you survive, the extent of the damage determines your future capacity or incapacity. Act fast.

Most heart attack deaths occur in the first two hours, yet studies found that many people wait four to six hours to get to an emergency room. Never ignore the warning signs of heart attack, including:

- Chest pain: an uncomfortable pressure, fullness, squeezing, or crushing feeling in the center of the chest that lasts two minutes or longer
- Severe pain that radiates to the shoulders, neck, arms (especially left arm), jaw, or top of the stomach
- Shortness of breath
- Paleness
- Sweating
- Rapid or irregular pulse
- Dizziness
- Fainting or loss of consciousness

Not all of these warning signs occur in every heart attack. Some people confuse heart attack symptoms with indigestion, a pulled muscle, or even a toothache. Women tend to experience more subtle symptoms – nausea, dizziness, sweating, jaw pain, fainting – rather than the classic chest pain. And some people, especially older people and diabetics, may not experience symptoms during a heart attack. (Only an electrocardiogram can reveal these so-called "silent heart attacks.") Two things these non-classic heart attacks had in common: the symptoms are unusual to the person and the symptoms are constant rather than coming and going.

If you suspect you may be experiencing a heart attack, get emergency medical help immediately. Doctors can prescribe a number of drugs that dissolve clots and reduce the oxygen demands of the heart, and these medications are most effective if given within one hour of the onset of a heart attack.

WOMEN AND MEN: HEART TO HEART

For decades, cardiovascular disease research involved only male subjects. More recent studies show that women aren't just small men. They have different cardiovascular risk profiles:

- After age 60, men and women have the same risk of heart disease – and one in four will die of cardiovascular disease. Before age 60, a woman's risk of having a heart attack is one in seventeen, compared to a one in five risk for men.[1]
- Heart attacks are more deadly in women. Thirty eight percent of women who have a heart attack die within a year, compared to 25 percent of men.[2]
- Women tend to take longer to seek medical care for a heart attack. They often have less severe symptoms, and they are less likely to experience the "classic" symptom of chest pain.
- Cholesterol abnormalities pose different risks in women and men. Elevated triglyceride levels are a significant predictor of heart disease in women (but not in men). In addition, elevated LDL cholesterol is a more significant risk factor for men than women.

Footnotes Appendix A

1 Bales, A.C. In search of lipid balance in older women. *Postgraduate Medicine*, 2000 Dec; 108 (7): 57-72.

2 American Heart Association, 2001 Women, heart disease and stroke statistics. http://www.americanheart.org/statistics/

APPENDIX B

More Good Books

Bland JS PhD and Benum SH. Genetic Nutritioneering: *How You can Modify Inherited Traits and Live a Longer, Healthier Life*. Keats Publishing: Los Angeles, CA, 1999

Bowden, Jonny. *Living the Low-Carb Life: From Atkins to the Zone Choosing the Diet That's Right for You*. Sterling, 2003

Brand-Miller J, Wolever T, Foster-Powell K, and Colaguiri S. *The New Glucose Revolution: The Authoritative Guide to the Glycemic Index*. Marlowe & Company: NY, 1996.

Cohen, Jay S. MD. *Over Dose: The Case Against the Drug Companies*. Penguin Putnam: NY, 2001.

Cooke, John P. MD PhD and Zimmer, Judith. *The Cardiovascular Cure: How to Strengthen Your Self Defense Against Heart Attack and Stroke*. Broadway Books: NY, 2002.

Critser, Greg. *Fat Land: How Americans Became the Fattest People in the World*. Houghton Mifflin Company: NY, 2003

Furey, Matt. *Combat Training: Functional Exercises for Fitness and Combat Sports*. Matt Furey Enterprises: Tampa, FL 2000.

Eades MR, MD and Eades MD, MD. *The Protein Power LifePlan*. Warner Books: New York, 2000.

Lyman F. with Merzer G. *Mad Cowboy: Plain Truth from the Cattle Rancher Who Won't Eat Meat*. Scribner: NY 1998.

McCully, Kilmer S MD and McCully, Martha. *The Heart Revolution: The Extraordinary Discovery That Finally Laid the Cholesterol Myth to Rest and Put Good Food Back on the Table.* HarperCollins: NY, 1999.

Mercola, Joseph MD with Levy, Alison Rose. *The No-Grain Diet: Conquer Carbohydrate Addiction and Stay Slim for Life.* Dutton: NY, 2003.

Natow, Annette B, PhD RD and Heslin, Jo-Ann, MA RD. *The Antioxidant Vitamin Counter.* Pocket Books: NY, 1994.

Pavel. *The Naked Warrior: Master the Secrets of the Super-Strong – Using Bodyweight Exercises Only.* DragonDoor Publications: St. Paul, MN, 2004

Ravnskov, Uff MD PhD. *The Cholesterol Myths.* New Trends Publishing: Washington, DC, 2000.

Robinson, Jo. *Why Grassfed is Best.* Vashon Island Press: WA, 2000.

Schlosser, Eric. *Fast Food Nation: The dark side of the all-American meal.* HarperCollins Publishers: NY, 2001.

Schmid, Ronald F. MD. *Traditional Foods Are Your Best Medicine,* Healing Arts Press: Rochester, VT, 1997.

Sears, Barry MD. *The Omega Rx Zone: The Miracle of the New High-Dose Fish Oil.* Regan Books, 2002

Sinatra, Stephen T. MD. *The Coenzyme Q10 Phenomenon.* Lowell House: Los Angeles, CA, 1998.

Sinatra, Stephen T MD and Sinatra J MSN. *Lower Your Blood Pressure in Eight Weeks.* Ballantine Books: NY, 2003.

Whitaker, Julian MD. *Reversing Heart Disease.* Warner Books: NY, 2000.

Willett, Walter MD. *Eat, Drink, and Be Healthy.* Fireside: NY, 2002.

APPENDIX C

Study Summaries

Dietary Fat and Heart Disease

Brehm BJ, Seeley RJ, Daniels SR, and D'Allessio DA. A random-ized trial comparing a very low carbohydrate diet and a calorie restricted low-fat diet on bodyweight and cardiovascular risk factors in healthy women. *Journal of Clinical Endocrine* Metabo-lism. 2003 Apr; 88(4):1617-1623.

53 healthy, obese (BMI=33.6) women were randomized to either (a) very low carbohydrate diet or (b) calorie restricted diet with 30% of the calories as fat. Researchers assessed metabolic measures at 3 and 6 months. The very low carbohydrate group lost more weight (8.5 pounds vs. 3.9 pounds). Blood pressure, lipids, glucose and insulin improved in both groups. Conclusion: A very low carbo-hydrate diet is more effective than a low-fat diet for weight loss and is not associated with heart risk factors.

Deming DM, Boileau AC, Lee CM and Erdman JW Jr. Amount of dietary fat and type of soluble fiber independently modulate postabsorptive conversion of beta-carotene to vitamin A in mongolian gerbils. *Journal of Nutrition.* 2000 Nov; 130(11): 2789-2796.

Current dietary guidelines recommend a decrease in fat intake and an increase in fiber consumption. This animal study tested a variety of diets on Mongolian gerbils to see variations in fat and fiber affected the absorption of Vitamin A. Results: betacarotine IS affected by dietary fat level and type of soluble fiber, compro-mising the absorption of betacarotine into Vitamin A.

Gradek WQ, Harris MT, Yahia N, et al. Polyunsaturated fatty acids acutely suppress antibodies to malondialdehyde-modified lipoproteins in patients with vascular disease. *American Journal of Cardiology.* **2004 Apr 1; 93(7);881-885.**

The study was designed to find out if meals high in fat reduce the antibodies to LDL. Though the number was small (10), the study was rigorously designed, and found that polyunsaturated fatty acids (PUFA) may indeed be a major source of oxidized lipids in the blood of patients with patients of arteriosclerosis. PUFA are acting as an anti-inflammatory in the body.

Hooper L, Summerbell CD, Higgins JPT, et al. Reduced or modified dietary fat for preventing cardiovascular disease. *The Cochrane Library.* **No. 2, 2004.**

The review covered 27 studies reporting on 1,144 subjects to see whether reduction or modification of dietary fat improved total cholesterol levels or had other effects on cardiovascular risk factors. Findings showed no significant effect on mortality, some protection from cardiovascular mortality, and significant protection from cardiovascular problems. Since the studies did not distinguish the types of fat, there is no conclusion that reducing dietary fat prevents cardiovascular disease.

Knopp RH, Walden CE, Retzlaff BM, et al. Long-term cholesterol-lowering effects of 4 fat-restricted diets in hypercholesterolemic and combined hyperlipidemic men. The Dietary Alternatives Study. Journal of the American Medical Association. 1997 (Nov 12; 278(18): 1509-1515.

444 men, separated into groups depending on levels of LDL and triglycerides, were randomized to 4 different diets containing either 30%, 26%, 22% or 18% fat, which they followed for a year. Results showed that moderate restriction of dietary fat (22-26%) had meaningful and sustained reduction in LDL levels of the participants. Extreme reduction of fat (18%) did not offer further advantage.

Mozaffarian D, Pischon T, Hankinson SE, et al. Dietary intake of trans fatty acids and systemic inflammation in women. *American Journal of Clinical Nutrition.* 2004 Apr; 79(4):606-612.

Trans fatty acid (TFA) intake predicts risks of coronary artery disease and diabetes. 823 healthy women participated in this study. Statistical analysis suggests that serum lipid concentrations may be partly mediated by effects of TFA. Researchers concluded that TFA intake is positively associated with markers of systemic inflammation in women.

Venkatraman JT, Leddy J, and Pendergast D. Dietary fats and immune status in athletes: clinical implications. *Medicine and Science of Sports Exercise*, 2000 Jul; 32(7Suppl):S389-95.

Studies have shown that a low-fat, high carbohydrate diet (15% fat, 65% carbohydrates) typically eaten by athletes increases inflammatory and decreases immune factors, depresses anti-oxidants and negatively affects blood lipoprotein ratios. Increasing the dietary fat intake of athletes to 42% does not negatively affect immune competency or blood lipoproteins, whereas it improves endurance exercise performance for cyclists and runners.

Warensjo E, Jansson JH, Berglund L, et al. Estimated intake of milk fat is negatively associated with cardiovascular risk factors and does not increase the risk of a first acute myocardial infarction. A prospective case-control study. British Journal of Nutrition. 2004 Apr; 91(4):635-642.

Researchers set out to see if the saturated fatty acids (SFA) in milk was associated with cardiovascular disease. 78 patients and 156 controls were matched for age, sex, and geographic region. Although there seemed to be a negative association between milk-fat intake and serum lipids, once clinical risk factors were calculated in, there was no relationship between SFA and cardiovascular disease.

Wolf RL, Cauley, JA, Baker, CE, et al. Factors associated with calcium absorption efficiency in pre- and perimenopausal women. *American Journal of Clinical Nutrition*, 2000 Aug; 72(2):466-471.

442 healthy pre- and perimenopausal women were studied for their

absorption of calcium. The study showed that calcium absorption averaged 35%, with a range of 17-58%. The amount of dietary fat consumed relative to fiber appears to have an important role in determining the differences in calcium absorption.

Cholesterol and Heart Disease

Auer W, Eiber A, Hostkorn E, et al. Hypertension and hyperlipi-daemia: Garlic helps in mild cases. *British Journal of Clini-cal Practical Supplements*. 1990 Aug; 69:3-6.

47 patients with mild hypertension took part in a trial where they either received garlic powder or a placebo for 12 weeks. Researchers moni-tored blood pressure and blood lipids at 4, 8, and 12 weeks. Sig-nificant differences were found. In the group taking garlic, their average dias-tolic (lower) blood pressure dropped from 102 to 89, and both choles-terol and triglycerides were significantly reduced. No significant changes occurred in the placebo group.

Castelli WP. Cholesterol and lipids in the risk of coronary artery disease-- the Framingham Heart Study. *Canadian Journal of Cardiology*. 1998 July; 4 Suppl A:5A-10A.

A screening process based on the high blood pressure campaign started in the 1970s aims at identifying people with elevated cholesterol so mea-sures can be taken to prevent heart attacks. Data from the 35 years of the Framingham Heart Study have shown that factors other than total or LDL cholesterol must be considered when evaluating coronary artery disease (CAD). The best simple test for predicting CAD is the ratio of total:HDL cholesterol.

Furman B, Rosenblat M, Hayek T, et al. Ginger extract consump-tion reduces plasma cholesterol, inhibits LDL oxidation and attenuates develop-ment of atherosclerosis in atherosclerotic apolipoprotein E-deficient mice. *Journal of Nutrition*. 2000 May; 130(5): 1124-1131.

Researchers assumed that consumption of nutrients rich in antioxidants were associated with reduced development of atherosclerosis.

Researchers worked with 60 mice divided into 3 groups – placebo, 25mcg ginger and 250mcg ginger. They found that adding ginger to the diet of the mice did, indeed, reduce the development of atherosclerosis and was associated with significant reduction in LDL cholesterol levels.

Ghirlanda G, Oradei A, Manto A, et al. Evidence of plasma CoQ10-lowering effect of HMG-CoA reductase inhibitors: a double-blind, placebo-controlled study. *Journal of Clinical Pharmacology*, **1993 Mar; 33(3): 226-229.**
Researchers studied 10 healthy volunteers and 30 patients with high cholesterol who took statin drugs or placebo. Researchers studied pre- and post-lab results for 10 measures. CoQ10 was reduced by 40% after the treatment. CoQ10 is essential for the production of energy and has antioxidant properties. Reducing CoQ10 in the human body may cause membrane alteration and cellular damage.

Gordon T, Castelli WP, Hjortland MC, et al. High density lipoprotein as a protective factor against coronary heart disease. The Framingham Study. *American Journal of Medicine,* **1977 May; 62(5):707-714.**
2,815 adults took part in the Framingham Study from 1969 to 1971. During that time 142 people developed coronary heart disease (CHD). Researchers obtained baseline and follow-up lipid values. Low HDL was the most potent risk factor for CHD, with LDL having a weaker association. Triglycerides were associated with CHD only in women.

Graham IM, Daly LE, Refsum HM, et al. Plasma homocysteine as a risk factor for vascular disease: The European Concerted Action Project. *Journal of the American Medical Association.* **1997 June 22; 277(22): 1775-1781.**
Nineteen centers in 9 European countries studied 750 people with vascular disease and 800 health people. An increased homocysteine level gave an independent risk of vascular disease similar to that of smoking or high cholesterol. When high homocysteine level was combined with smoking or high cholesterol, the odds of vascular disease increased enormously. Researchers suggest doing studies of the effects of vitamins

to reduce homocysteine levels and therefore vascular disease risk.

Hunninghake DB, Maki KC, Kwiterovich PO Jr, et al. Incorporation of lean red meat into a National Cholesterol Education Program Step I diet: a long-term randomized clinical trial in free-living persons with hypercholesterolemia. *Journal of the American College of Nutrition.* **2000 Jun; 19(3):351-360.**

145 subjects with high cholesterol levels were divided into 2 groups eating 6 ounces daily of either red meat (beef, veal or pork) or white meat (poultry or fish) for 36 weeks. The results showed that both diets were effective in lowering LDL cholesterol and increasing HDL concentrations.

Jenkins DJ, Kendall CW, Marchie A, et al. Effects of a dietary portfolio of cholesterol-lowering foods vs. Lovastatin on serum lipids and C-reactive protein. *Journal of the American Medical Association.* **2003 Jul; 290(4):502-510.**

46 patients with high cholesterol were divided into 3 groups: control (low-fat diet), statin (+low-fat) and dietary (high protein and fiber). Each group followed their protocol for 30 days. Pre- and post-blood tests showed that both the statin and dietary groups did much better than the control group. The researchers concluded that varying dietary components increased the effectiveness of diet as a treatment of high cholesterol.

Knopp RH, Walden CE, Retzlaff BM, et al. Long-term cholesterol-lowering effects of 4 fat-restricted diets in hypercholesterolemic and combined hyperlipidemic men. The Dietary Alternatives Study. *Journal of the American Medical Association.* **1997 (Nov 12; 278(18): 1509-1515.**

444 men were separated into groups depending on their levels of LDL and triglycerides. These groups were randomized to 4 different diets, containing 30%, 26%, 22% or 18% fat, which they followed for a year. Results showed that moderate restriction of dietary fat (22-26%) had meaningful and sustained reduction in LDL levels of the participants. Extreme reduction of fat (18%) did not offer further advantage.

Krumholz HM, Seeman TE, Merrill SS, et al. Lack of association between cholesterol and coronary heart disease mortality and morbidity and all-cause mortality in persons older than 70 years. *Journal of the American Medical Association.* **1994 Nov 2; 272(17):1335.**

997 subjects, more than 70 years old, participated in the study from 1988 to 1992. Researchers found that total cholesterol and low HDL were not associated with a significantly higher rate of all-cause mortality, coronary heart disease or hospitalization for heart attack or angina in people of 70 years of age.

Mendall M, Patel P, Ballam L, et al. C-reactive protein and its relation to cardiovascular risk factors: a population based cross sectional study. *British Medical Journal,* **1996 Apr 27; 312(7038):1061-1065.**

303 men (aged 50-69) took part in the study. Increasing age, smoking, symptoms of chronic bronchitis, infections and body mass index were all associated with raised concentrations of C-reactive protein, which was also associated with cholesterol, triglyceride, and glucose values. Researchers concluded that the body's response to inflammation may play an important part in influencing the progression of atherosclerosis.

Ravnoskov U. Cholesterol lowering trials in coronary heart disease: frequency of citation and outcome. *British Journal of Medicine.* **1991 July 4; 305(6844):15-19.**

Researcher reviewed 22 controlled cholesterol lowering trials to verify the claim that lowering cholesterol values prevents coronary heart disease. Researcher found that those trials which to be supportive of lowering cholesterol were cited 6 times more often than trials were did not support this position. Therefore, claims that lowering cholesterol prevents coronary heart disease are based only on the preferential citation of certain supportive trials.

Ridker PM, Rifai N, Rose L, et al. Comparison of C-reactive protein and low-density lipoprotein cholesterol levels in the predication of first cardiovascular events. *New England Journal of Medicine.* **2002 Nov 14; 347(20):1557-1565.**

Ridker PM, Rifai N, Rose L, et al. Comparison of C-reactive protein and low-density lipoprotein cholesterol levels in the predication of first cardiovascular events. *New England Journal of Medicine.* 2002 Nov 14; 347(20):1557-1565.

27,939 healthy women provided baseline measures for C-reactive protein (CRP) and LDL, and were followed for 8 years. The baseline levels of the two measures were strongly related to the incidence of cardiovascular event, even when adjusting for age, smoking, diabetes, and blood pressure. CRP is a stronger predictor of cardiovascular problems than LDL cholesterol and adds important prognostic data to the risk of cardiovascular events.

Williams PT, Stefanick MR, Vranizan KM and Wood PD. The effects of weight loss by exercise or by dieting on plasma high-density lipoprotein (HDL) levels in men with low, intermediate, and normal-to-high HDL at baseline. *Metabolism.* 1994 Jul; 43(7): 917-924.

130 men, aged 30 to 59, were randomized for 1 year to lose weight by exercise, by caloric restriction, or to make no effort to lose weight. Baseline HDL levels were documented. The increase in HDL cholesterol levels was significantly greater in the men who had low HDL at baseline.

The Lipid Research Clinics Coronary Primary Prevention Trial results. I. Reduction in incidence of coronary heart disease. *Journal of the American Medical Association.* 1984 Jan 20; 251(3):351-364.

Researchers followed 3,806 middle-aged men with high cholesterol levels for 7 years. Half the men took a bile acid sequestrant cholestryramine resin and the other half took a placebo; all participants followed a moderate cholesterol lowering diet. The risk of death from all causes was not significantly reduced in the drug-taking group. However men at high risk of coronary heart disease because of high LDL levels experienced lower incidence of coronary heart disease by lowering their LDL levels.

Drugs and Heart Disease

Crouse JR 3rd, Byington RP, Bond MG, et al. Pravastatin, lipids, and atherosclerosis in the carotid arteries (PLAC-II). *American Journal of Cardiology*. 1995 Mar 1; 75(7):455-459.

Researchers randomized 151 coronary patients meeting certain inclusion criteria to placebo or pravastatin and treated them for 3 years. Results showed non-significant reduction in carotid artery thickness, though blood lipid levels decreased and there was a significant decrease in fatal and nonfatal coronary events.

Ghirlanda G, Oradei A, Manto A, et al. Evidence of plasma CoQ10-lowering effect of HMG-CoA reductase inhibitors: a double-blind, placebo-controlled study. *Journal of Clinical Pharmacology*, 1993 Mar; 33(3): 226-229.

Researchers studied 10 healthy volunteers and 30 patients with high cholesterol who took statin drugs or placebo. Researchers studied pre- and post-lab results for 10 measures. CoQ10 was reduced by 40% after the treatment. CoQ10 is essential for the production of energy and has antioxidant properties. Reducing CoQ10 in the human body may cause membrane alteration and cellular damage.

Grimm RH Jr, Leon AS, Hunninghake DB, et al. Effects of thiazide diuretics on plasma lipids and lipoproteins in mildly hypertensive patients: a double-blind controlled trial. *Annals of Internal Medicine*. 1981 Jan; 94(1):7-11.

Compared to baseline, both total cholesterol and triglycerides rose with treatment by diuretics. A cholesterol-lowering diet largely prevents this increase. Because the effects of diuretics may cancel part of the potential benefit of blood pressure control, physicians should prescribe a cholesterol-lowering diet and periodically monitor patients' blood lipid levels.

Grossman E, Ironi AN and Messerli FH. Comparative tolerability profile of hypertensive crisis treatments. *Drug Safety.* 1998 Aug; 19(2):99-122.

Hypertensive crisis is defined as a severe elevation in blood pressure. While the efficacy of available treatments seems similar, the underlying mechanism of action and potential for adverse effects should guide choice. The researchers list 14 different hypertensive medications and the different situations in which each should be used. They recommend that patients with hypertensive emergencies be treated to lower the mean arterial pressure by 25% over the initial 2-4 hours with the most specific hypertensive agent.

Kuhn M. Nitrates. *AACN Clinical Issues in Critical Care Nursing.* 1992 May; 3(2):409-422.

Nitrates have been used for the past 130 years to treat and control symptoms of angina. Nitrates work by directly relaxing smooth muscle in vessels, thereby causing generalized dilation. This review covers indications for nitrate use, usefulness of nitrates and nursing implications.

Lewis BE and McDonough K. Dyslipidemia treatment among patients with coronary artery disease in a managed care organization. *American Journal of Health-System Pharmacy.* 2004 May 15; 61(10);1032-1038.

A review of records in a large managed care organization evaluated patients with coronary artery disease (CAD) to evaluate the effectiveness of statin prescriptions. Reviewers found that while 39.8% of the patients received a statin, only 24% of them were tested for LDL. Of those patients who received statins, 44.5% achieved the LDL goal level. However, of the patients who were tested, but did not receive statins, 29.8% also achieved the LDL goal level.

Manktelow B, Gillies C and Potter JF. Interventions in the management of serum lipids for preventing stroke recurrence (Cochrane Review). *The Cochrane Library.* 2004: 2.

Five studies involving 1,700 patients were included. The medicines included were Clofibrate, Pravastatin and Conjugated Oestrogen.

Results showed no evidence of a difference in stroke recurrence between the treatment and placebo groups. There was also no evidence that this intervention reduced the odds of all-cause mortality.

Pahor M, Psaty BM, Alderman MH, et al. Health outcomes associated with calcium antagonists compared with other first-line antihypertensive therapies: meta-analysis of randomized controlled trials. *Lancet.* **2000 Dec 9; 356(9246):1949-1954.**

In reviewing 9 randomised controlled trials included 27,743 patients, calcium antagonists were inferior to other types of antihypertensive drugs as first-line agents in reducing the risks of several major complications of hypertension. Based on these data, the longer-acting calcium antagonists cannot be recommended as first-line therapy for hypertension.

Psaty B, Heckbert SR, Koepsell TD, et al. The risk of myocardial infarction associated with antihypertensive drug therapies. *Journal of the American Medical Association.* **1995 Aug 23; 274(8):620-625.**

623 people who had a heart attack and 2,032 controls who were being treated for hypertension were studied for 4-7 years. Analysis of medications showed that there was an increased risk (60%) of heart attack among users of calcium channel blockers, as opposed to users of diuretics or beta-blockers. Researchers recommended that diuretics and beta blockers be used as first-line agents in hypertension, rather than calcium channel blockers.

Roten L, Shcoenenberger RA, Krohenbuyl S, Schlienger RG. Rhabdomyolysis in association with simvastatin and amiodarone. *Annals of Pharmacotherapy.* **2004 June; 38(6):978-981.**

A patient experienced severe myopathy associated with concomitant simvastatin and amiodarone therapy. Myopathy is a rare, but potentially severe, adverse reaction associated with statins. Physicians should avoid the concomitant use of these two drugs or eliminate the statins to decrease the risk of statin-associated myopathy.

Telfox, HT, et al. Conflict of interest in the debate over calcium-channel antagonists. *New England Journal of Medicine.* 1998 Jan 8; 338(2):101-106.

Physician's financial relationships with the pharmaceutical industry are controversial because such relationships may pose a conflict of interest. Researchers reviewed medical literature from March 1995 to September 1996 for articles examining the safety of calcium-channel antagonists. Results showed that authors who supported the use of calcium-channel antagonists were significantly more likely (96%) to have financial relationships with manufacturers of calcium-channel antagonists.

Willcox SM, Himmelstein DU and Wooldhandler S. Inappropriate drug prescribing for the community-dwelling elderly. *Journal of the American Medical Association.* 1994 Jul 27; 272(4):292-296.

Researchers found that physicians prescribe potentially inappropriate medications for nearly 25% of all older people living in the community, placing them at risk of drug adverse effects such as cognitive impairment and sedation. Although most previous strategies for improving drug prescribing for the elderly have focused on nursing homes, broader educational and regulatory initiatives are needed.

Yusuf S, Sleight P, Pogue J, et al. Effects of an angiotensin-converting-enzyme inhibitor, rampipril, on cardiovascular events in high-risk patients. The Heart Outcomes Prevention Evaluation Study Investigators. *New England Journal of Medicine.* 2000 Jan 20; 342(3):145-153.

9,297 patients (55 or older) with evidence of vascular disease or diabetes were randomly assigned to receive ramipril or placebo for 5 years. Ramipril inhibits angiotensin-converting-enzyme (ACE). Ramipril significantly reduced the rates of death, myocardial infection, and stroke in a broad range of high-risk patients.

Inflammation and Heart Disease

Beck J, Garcia R, Heiss G, et al. Periodontal disease and cardiovascular disease. *Journal of Periodontistry* 1996 Oct; 67(10 Sup):1123-1137.

1,147 veterans, treated for periodontal disease between 1968 and 1971, were also checked for cardiovas-cular disease. Researchers hypothesized that periodontal disease represents a risk factor for atherosclerosis due to an underlying inflammatory response trait. Adjusting for established cardiovascular risk factors, researchers found that veterans with periodontal disease were 1.5 times more likely to have coronary heart disease, 1.9 times more likely to die of coronary heart disease, and 2.8 times more likely to have a stroke.

Church T, Barlow CE, Earnest CP, et al. Associations between cardiorespiratory fitness and C-reactive protein in men. *Arteriosclerosis and Thrombosis: Journal of Vascular Biology.* 2002 Nov 1; 22(11):1869-1879.

Researchers studied 722 men to examine the association between cardiorespiratory fitness and C-reactive protein (CRP) levels, with adjustments for weight and 9 other variables. Conclusion: Cardiorespiratory fitness levels were inversely associated with CRP levels. In other words, men with higher levels of CRP had the lowest levels of cardiorespiratory fitness, and men with lower levels of CRP had the highest levels of cardiorespiratory fitness.

Fichtischerer S, Rosenberger G, Walter DH, et al. Elevated C-reactive protein levels and impaired endothelial vasoreactivity in patients with coronary artery disease. *Circulation.* 2000 Aug 29; 102(9):1000-1006.

Researchers tested 60 adult males with coronary artery disease (CAD) for classic risk factors of CAD. Elevated C-reactive protein (CRP) levels were a statistically significant predictor of blunted vasodilator capacity. Elevated CRP serum levels as a risk factor might provide an important clue to link systemic marker inflammation to atherosclerotic disease progression.

Genco R. Periodontal disease and cardiovascular disease: epidemiology and possible mechanisms. Journal of American Dental Association. 2002 Jun; 133 Suppl:14S-22S.

The authors reviewed longitudinal, case control and cross-sectional studies of the relationship between periodontal and cardiovascular disease. The evidence shows that there is a moderate association between the two disease processes – periodontal infection may, indeed, be a contributing risk factor for heart disease.

Graham IM, Daly LE, Refsum HM, et al. Plasma homocysteine as a risk factor for vascular disease: The European Concerted Action Project. *Journal of the American Medical Association.* **1997 June 22; 277(22):1775-1781.**

Nineteen centers in 9 European countries studied 750 people with vascular disease and 800 healthy people. An increased homocysteine level gave an independent risk of vascular disease similar to that of smoking or high cholesterol. When high homocysteine level was combined with smoking or high cholesterol, the odds of vascular disease increased enormously. Researchers suggest doing studies of the effects of vitamins to reduce homocysteine levels and therefore vascular disease risk.

Hunt PA, Hunt KE, Susiarjo M, et al. Bisphenol a exposure causes meiotic aneuploidy in the female mouse. *Current Biology.* **2003 Apr 1; 13(7):546-553.**

While conducting another experiment, researchers realized that the mice had been compromised by exposure to bisphenol A (BPA) – an estrogenic compound widely used in the production of plastics and epoxy resins. They replicated the experimental conditions and found that both the initial inadvertent exposure and subsequent experimental studies suggest that BPA powerfullu causes chromosome damage.

Kanauchi M, Tsujimoto N and Hashimoto T. Advanced glycation end products in nondiabetic patients with coronary artery disease. *Diabetes Care.* **2001 (Sep), 24(9): 1620-1623.**

48 non-diabetic patients with history of chest pain or suspected coronary artery disease (CAD) were tested in a number of ways. Sophisticated statistical techniques showed that there was a definite relationship between advanced glycation end products (AGEs) and the severity of CAD in non-diabetic patients. Measurement of AGE concentrations may be predictive of vascular damage.

Mendall M, Patel P, Ballam L, et al. C-reactive protein and its relation to cardiovascular risk factors: a population based cross sectional study. *British Medical Journal,* 1996 Apr 27; 312(7038):1061-1065.

303 men (aged 50-69) took part in the study. Increasing age, smoking, symptoms of chronic bronchitis, infections and body mass index were all associated with raised concentrations of C-reactive protein, which was also associated with cholesterol, triglyceride, and glucose values. Researchers concluded that the body's response to inflammation may play an important part in influencing the progression of atherosclerosis.

Ridker PM, Rifai N, Rose L, et al. Comparison of C-reactive protein and low-density lipoprotein cholesterol levels in the predication of first cardiovascular events. *New England Journal of Medicine.* 2002 Nov 14; 347(20):1557-1565.

27,939 healthy women provided baseline measures for C-reactive protein (CRP) and LDL, and were followed for 8 years. The baseline levels of the two measures were strongly related to the incidence of cardiovascular event, even when adjusting for age, smoking, diabetes, and blood pressure. CRP is a stronger predictor of cardiovascular problems than LDL cholesterol and adds important prognostic data to the risk of cardiovascular events.

Ridker PM, Hennekens CH, Buring JE and Rifai N. C-reactive protein and other markers of inflammation in the reduction of cardiovascular disease in women. *New England Journal of Medicine.* 2000 Mar 23; 342(12):836-843.

28,263 healthy, post-menopausal women were followed for 3 years to assess the risk of cardiovascular events associated with base-line levels of markers of inflammation. Of the 12 markers measured, C-reactive protein (CRP) was the strongest predictor of the risk of cardiovascular events. Even when LDL levels were below 130 CRP was a strong predictor of heart problems. CRP levels should be included when screening lipid levels to provide an improved method of identifying persons at risk for cardiovascular events.

Ridker PM, Cushman M, Stampfer MJ, et al. Inflammation, aspirin, and the risk of cardiovascular disease in apparently healthy men. *New England Journal of Medicine.* 1997 Apr 3; 336(14): 973-979.

543 healthy men were followed for 8 years. The groups were randomly assigned to receive aspirin or placebo. Baseline C-reactive protein (CRP) was higher in those who had subsequent heart problems. The reduction in risk of heart attack associated with aspirin was directly related to the level of CRP, raising the possibility that anti-inflammatory agents (ie, aspirin) may have clinical benefits in preventing cardiovascular disease.

Siegel AJ, Lewandrowski EL, Chun KY, et al. Changes in cardiac markers including B-natriuretic peptide in runners after the Boston Marathon. *American Journal of Cardiology.* 2001 Oct 15; 88(8): 920-923.

From 1996 to 2001 Boston Marathon runners provided blood samples before and after the race. Post-race results showed an imbalance in clotting and inflammatory factors known to set the stage for heart attack. Though none of the marathon runners suffered heart trouble during or after the marathon, researchers warn that high-risk individuals with high blood pressure, diabetes or other chronic conditions may want to avoid running in marathons.

Stampfer M, Malinow MR, Willett WC, et al. A prospective study of plasma homocyst(e)ine and risk of myocardial infarction in US physicians. *Journal of the American Medical Association.* 1992 Aug 19; 268(7):877-881.

14,916 men, aged 40 to 84, without prior heart attack or stroke, provided baseline blood samples and were followed for 5 years. 271 men subsequently developed heart attacks and were analyzed for homocystein levels. Moderately high levels of plasma homocystein are associated with subsequent risk of heart attack, independent of other risk factors. High levels of homocystein levels can be easily treated with vitamin supplements.

Vlassara H, Cai W, Crandall J, et al. Inflammatory mediators are induced by dietary glycotoxins, a major risk factor for diabetic angiopathy. *Proceedings of National Academy of Science USA.* 2002 Nov 26; 99(24):15596-15601.

37 diabetic subjects followed specific diets for 6 weeks and multiple blood samples were drawn. It was found that dietary AGEs (advanced glycation end products) promote inflammatory mediators, leading to tissue injury. Therefore, restriction of dietary AGEs suppress these effects.

Yeargans G and Seidler NW. Carnosine promotes the heat denaturation of glycated protein. Biochemical Biophysical Research Community. 2003 Jan 3; 300(1):75-80.

Glycation alters protein structure and decreases biological activity. Carnosine prevents glycation and may also play a role in the disposal of glycated protein. Carnosine may promote hydration during heat denaturation of glycated protein.

Food for Heart Health

Brehm BJ, Seeley RJ, Daniels SR, and D'Allessio DA. A random-ized trial comparing a very low carbohydrate diet and a calorie restricted low-fat diet on bodyweight and cardiovascular risk factors in healthy women. Journal of Clinical Endocrine Metabo-lism. 2003 Apr; 88(4):1617-1623.

53 healthy, obese (BMI=33.6) women were randomized to either (a) very low carbohydrate diet or (b) calorie restricted diet with 30% of the calories as fat. Researchers assessed metabolic measures at 3 and 6 months. The very low carbohydrate group lost more weight (8.5 pounds vs. 3.9 pounds). Blood pressure, lipids, glucose and insulin improved in both groups over the course of the study. Conclusion: A very low carbohydrate diet is more effective than a low-fat diet for short-term weight loss and is not associated with cardiovascular risk factors.

Cordain L, Miller JB, Eaton SB, et al. Plant-animal subsistence ratios and macronutrient energy estimations in worldwide hunter-gatherer diets. *The American Journal of Clinical Nutrition.* 2000 Mar; 71(3); 682-692.

Researchers reconstructed the traditional diet of pre-agricultural humans, incorporating ethno-graphic compilation of plant-to-animal subsistence patterns of hunter-gatherers to estimate likely dietary intakes. Analysis showed that most hunter-gatherers consumed approximately 19-35% protein and 22-40% carbohydrates, whereas modern US adults eat approximately 16% protein and 49% carbohydrates.

Deming DM, Boileau AC, Lee CM and Erdman JW Jr. Amount of dietary fat and type of soluble fiber independently modulate postabsorptive conversion of beta-carotene to vitamin A in mongolian gerbils. *Journal of Nutrition.* 2000 Nov; 130(11): 2789-2796.

Current dietary guidelines recommend a decrease in fat intake and an increase in fiber consumption. This animal study tested a variety of diets on Mongolian gerbils to see variations in fat and fiber affected the absorption of Vitamin A. Results: betacarotine IS affected by dietary fat level and type of soluble fiber, compro-mising the absorption of betac-arotine into Vitamin A.

French P, Stanton C, Lawless F, et al. Fatty acid composition, including conjugated linoleic acid, of intramuscular fat from steers offered grazed grass, grass silage, or concentrate-based diets. *Journal of Animal Science,* 2000 Nov; 78(11):2849-2855.

Fifty steers were divided into five groups and given different dietary treatments. The concentration of polyunsaturated fatty acids in intra-muscular fat was highest in those eating only grazed grass – and the concentration of saturated fatty acids was the lowest. The implication for human health is that it is best to eat grass fed cows.

Gutierrez M, Akhavan M, Jovanovic L and Peterson CM. Utility of a short-term 25% carbohydrate diet on improving glycemic control in type 2 diabetes mellitus. *Journal of the American College of Nutrition.* 1998 Dec; 17(6):595-600.

Researchers studied 28 subjects with type 2 diabetes, divided into diet alone or diet comprised of 25% carbohydrates. The conclusion was that a low carbohydrate, reduced-calorie diet had beneficial effects in type 2 diabetic subjects who had failed either diet or insulin therapy. The low carbohydrate diet may reduce the need for insulin therapy.

He K, Rimm EB, Merchant A, et al. Fish consumption and risk of stroke in men. *Journal of the American Medical Association,* **2002 Dec 25; 288(24):3130-3136.**
Researchers studied 43,671 men, aged 40-75 years, over a period of 12 years. 608 men (14%) had strokes during the 12 year follow-up period. Researchers found that men who ate fish less than once a month were most likely to have strokes; men who ate fish 1-3 times per month achieved the greatest benefit.

Hunninghake DB, Maki KC, Kwiterovich PO Jr, et al. Incorporation of lean red meat into a National Cholesterol Education Program Step I diet: a long-term randomized clinical trial in free-living persons with hypercholesterolemia. *Journal of the American College of Nutrition.* **2000 Jun; 19(3):351-360.**
145 subjects with high cholesterol levels were divided into 2 groups eating 6 ounces daily of either red meat (beef, veal or pork) or white meat (poultry or fish) for 36 weeks. The results showed that both diets were effective in lowering LDL cholesterol and increasing HDL concentrations.

Hunt PA, Hunt KE, Susiarjo M, et al. Bisphenol a exposure causes meiotic aneuploidy in the female mouse. Current Biology. 2003 April 1; 13(7):546-553.
Researchers working with mice found that exposure to BPA, widely used in the production of polycarbonate plastics and epoxy resins, caused problems in their reproductive process.

Jenkins DJ, Kendall CW, Marchie A, et al. Effects of a dietary portfolio of cholesterol-lowering foods vs. Lovastatin on serum lipids and C-reactive protein. *Journal of the American Medical Association.* 2003 Jul; 290(4):502-510.

46 patients with high cholesterol were divided into 3 groups: control (low-fat diet), statin (+low-fat) and dietary (high protein and fiber). Each group followed their protocol for 30 days. Pre- and post-blood tests showed that both the statin and dietary groups did much better than the control group. The researchers concluded that varying dietary components increased the effectiveness of diet as a treatment of high cholesterol.

Knopp RH, Walden CE, Retzlaff BM, et al. Long-term cholesterol-lowering effects of 4 fat-restricted diets in hypercholesterolemic and combined hyperlipidemic men. The Dietary Alternatives Study. *Journal of the American Medical Association.* 1997 (Nov 12; 278(18): 1509-1515.

444 men were separated into groups depending on their levels of LDL and triglycerides. These groups were randomized to 4 different diets, containing 30%, 26%, 22% or 18% fat, which they followed for a year. Results showed that moderate restriction of dietary fat (22-26%) had meaningful and sustained reduction in LDL levels of the participants. Extreme reduction of fat (18%) did not offer further advantage.

Lijnen HR, Maquoi E, Morange P, et al. Nutritionally induced obesity is attenuated in transgenic mice overexpressing plasminogen activator inhibitor-1. *Arteriosclerosis, Thrombosis and Vascular Biology.* 2003 Jan 1; 23(1):78-84.

This animal study had two groups of mice on either a standard diet or a high fat diet. After 15 weeks, researhers concluded that plasminogen activator inhibitor-1 causes nutritionally induced obesity. This may be related to modifications in fat tissue cellularity.

Mata Lopez P and Ortega RM. Omega-3 fatty acids in the prevention and control of cardiovascular disease. *European Journal of Clinical Nutrition.* 2003 Sep; 57 Suppl 1:S22-25.

Until recently, the dietetic criteria for preventing and controlling cardio-vascular disease has been restrictive in terms of fat intake. However, compliance is difficult and deficiencies might arise that negatively affect quality of life. Omega-3 fatty acids have been found to be beneficial with respect to cardiovascular disease. This paper discusses the sources of omega-3 fatty acids, their recommended consumption and possible mechanisms of action.

May PE, Barber A, D'Olimpio JT, et al. Reversal of cancer-wasting using oral supplementation with a combination of beta-hydroxy-beta-methylbu-tyrate, arginine and glutamine. *American Journal of Surgery.* **2002 April; 183(4):471-479.**

Researchers wanted to learn if specific nutrients related to protein syn-thesis would reverse the weight loss in advanced (Stage IV) cancer. 32 patients received 24 weeks of supplementation with beta-hydroxy-beta-methylbuyrate (HMB), arginine (ARG), and glutamine (GLN). This mixture proved effective in increasing fat-free mass in these patients, because the HMB slowed the rate of protein breakdown and ARG and GLN improved protein synthesis.

Mozaffarian D, Lemaitre RN, Juller LH, et al. Cardiac benefits of fish consumption may depend on the type of fish meal consumed: the Cardiovascular Health Study. *Circulation.* **2003 Mar 18; 107(10):1372-1377.**

3,910 adults over 65 years old participated in this study. Modest con-sumption of broiled or baked fish (not fried fish or fish sandwiches) was associated with lowering the risk of ischemic heart disease (IHD), especially arrhythmic IHD death. Cardiac benefits of fish consumption may vary depending on the type of fish consumed.

Pereira MA, Jacobs DR Jr, Van Horn L, et al. Dairy consumption, obe-sity, and the insulin resistance syndrome in young adults: the CARDIA Study. *Journal of the American Medical Association.* **2002 Apr 24; 287(16);2081-2089.**

3,157 adults, aged 18-30, were followed from 1985 through 1996. Researchers found that increased dairy consumption had a strong inverse association with insulin resistance syndrome among overweight adults and may reduce the risk of type 2 diabetes and cardiovascular disease.

Rabast U, Schonborn J and Kasper H. Dietetic treatment of obesity with low and high carbohydrate diets: comparative studies and clinical results. *International Journal of Obesity.* 1979; 3(3):201-211.
117 patients were randomized to either a low-carbohydrate diet or a high carbohydrate diet for 4 months. Patients showed much greater weight loss with the low-carbohydrate diet. 52 patients lost an average of 40 pounds and 65 patients lost an average of 29 pounds during the study.

Serra-Majem L, Ribas L, Tresserras R, et al. How could changes in diet explain changes in coronary heart disease? The Spanish paradox. *American Journal of Clinical Nutrition.* 1995 Jun; 61(6 Suppl):1351S-1359S.
Researchers reviewed trends in coronary heart disease (CHD) and strokes in Spain from 1966 to 1990, as well as changes in food consumption on a national level. Since 1976 CHD mortality has been decreasing. Trends in food consumption showed increases in intake of meat, dairy products, fish and fruit, but decreases in consumption of olive oil, sugar and foods rich in carbohydrates.

Vega-Lopez S, Vidal-Quintanar RL and Fernandez ML. Sex and hormonal status influence plasma lipid responses to psyllium. *American Journal of Clinical Nutrition.* 2001 Oct; 74(4):435-441.
Three groups of people were randomly assigned to a fiber supplement (15g psyllium per day) or a control. Psyllium lowered LDL by 7-9% without affecting HDL concentrations. However, the effect of psyllium on triacylglycerol differed between men and women – acting positively for men, negatively for post-menopausal women and neutrally for pre-menopausal women.

Waladkhani AR and Clemens MR. Effect of dietary phytochemicals on cancer development (review). *International Journal of Molecular Medicine.* 1998 Apr; 1(4):747-753.

Researchers found that phytochemicals can inhibit the beginning of cancer by scavenging DNA reactive agents, suppressing the abnormal proliferation of early lesions, and inhibit certain properties of cancer cells.

Wolf, RL, Cauley, JA, Baker, CE, et al. Factors associated with calcium absorption efficiency in pre- and perimenopausal women. *American Journal of Clinical Nutrition*, 2000 Aug; 72(2):466-471.

442 healthy pre- and perimenopausal women were studied for their absorption of calcium. The study showed that calcium absorption averaged 35%, with a range of 17-58%. Researchers found that lower dietary fat intake is significantly associated with lower calcium absorption values. Since calcium is already difficult for the body to absorb, anything that increases that difficulty is undesirable.

Exercise for Heart Health

Brose A, Parise G and Ternopolsy, MA. Creatine supplementation enhances isometric strength and body composition improvements following strength exercise training in older adults. *Journal of Gerontology Series A: Biological Science and Medical Science*, 2003 Jan; 58(1):11-19.

28 men and women over 65 years old participated in a resistance exercise program 3 days per week for 14 weeks. Half the group received creatine; the other half received a placebo. The study confirmed that supervised heavy resistance exercise training can safely increase muscle strength and functional capacity in older adults. The addition of creatine enhanced the increase in total and fat-free mass, and gains in several indices of isometric muscle strength.

DeBusk RF, Stenestrand U, Sheehan M and Haskell WL. Training effects of long versus short bouts of exercise in healthy subjects. American Journal of Cardiology. 1990 Apr 15; 65(15):1010-1013.

Eight week study separated 36 men into 2 groups: half (average age 45-57) completing 30 minutes of exercise daily and half (average age 46-58) completing three 10-minute bouts of exercise daily. Results showed that the multiple short bouts of moderate-intensity exercise produced a significant increase in peak oxygen uptake. Therefore, short bouts of exercise training may not only be more effective, but also more efficient in today's busy lifestyle.

Elam R, Hardin DH, Sutton RA, and Hagen L. Effects of arginine and ornithine on strength, lean body mass and urinary hydroxyproline in adult males. *Journal of Sports Medicine and Physical Fitness,* **1989 Mar; 29(1):52-56.**

22 adult men participated in a 5-week progressive strength training program, where half received amino acids, arginine and ornithine, and the other half received calcium and Vitamin C placebos. Conclusion: taking prescribed doses of arginine and ornithine in conjunction with a high intensity strength program increases total strength and lean body mass in a relatively short time. Arginine and ornithine aid in recovery from chronic stress by quelling tissue breakdown.

Fozard JL. Epidemiologists try many ways to show that physical activity is good for seniors' health and longevity. Review of special issue of the Journal of Aging and Physical Activity: The Evergreen Project. *Experimental Aging Research* **1999 Apr-Jun; 25(2):175-182.**

The Evergreen Project. Special issue of the Journal of Aging and Physical Activity. Volume 6(2); 1998. Original, multidisciplinary research articles from the Evergreen Longitudinal Study of Aging (Finland), based on the population of a midsized Finnish town over an 8 year period.

Halbert JA, Silagy CA, Finucane P, et al. The effectiveness of exercise training in lowering blood pressure: a meta-analysis of randomized controlled trial of 4 weeks or longer. Journal of Human Hypertension. 1997 Oct; 11(10):641-649.

Researchers set out to identify the features of an optimal exercise program to decrease blood pressure. 1,533 subjects (both normal and with hypertension) were separated into 3 types of exercise: aerobic, resistance training, or both aerobic and resistance training. They found that aerobic exercise had a clinically significant effect in reducing systolic and diastolic blood pressure. Increasing exercise frequency to more than 3 sessions per week did not have an additional impact.

Kraemer WJ, Hakkinen K, Newton RU, et al. Effects of heavy-resistance training on hormonal response patterns in younger vs. older men. *Journal of Applied Physiology.* **1999 Sep; 87(3): 982-992.**

Two groups of men (30 and 60 years old) participated in a 10-week strength-power training program. Researchers took multiple blood samples 15 times and analyzed the results. The older men demonstrated a significant increase in total testosterone along with significant decrease in resting cortisol. Both groups experienced an enhanced hormonal profile from the training program, but the response is different between the 2 groups.

LaStayo PC, Ewy GA, Pierotti DD, et al. The positive effects of negative work: increased muscle strength and decreased fall risk in a frail elderly population. *Journal of Gerontology and Biological Science and Medical Science.* **2003 May; 58(5):M419-424.**

21 frail, elderly subjects (mean age = 80 years) underwent 11 weeks of lower extremity resistance training, using 2 different types of exercises. The group which used a high-force eccentric ergometer experienced significant improvements in strength (60%), balance (7%) and stair descent ability (21%). Therefore, lower extremity resistance exercise can improve muscle structure and function in those with limited exercise tolerance.

Lee IM, Hsieh CC and Paffenbarger RS Jr. Exercise intensity and longevity in men. The Harvard Alumni Health Study. *Journal of the American Medical Association.* **1995 Apr 19; 273(15):1179-1184.**

17,321 Harvard University alumni were followed from 1962 through 1988, when these men completed physical activity questionnaires.

Mortality from all causes was 3,728 (21%). Researchers found an inverse relationship between total physical activity and mortality. Furthermore, vigorous activity was associated with greater longevity, though non-vigorous exercise has been shown to benefit other aspects of health.

Murphy M, Nevill A, Neville C, et al. Accumulating brisk walking for fitness, cardiovascular risk, and psychological health. *Medicine and Science in Sports and Exercise.* **2002 Sep; 34(9):1468-1474.**

21 adults, average age 44, participated in a 6 week program of walking in order to study the effects of different patterns of walking, risk factors for cardiovascular disease, and psychological well-being in previously sedentary adults. Researchers concluded that 3 short bouts (10 minutes) of brisk waking in a day were at least as effective as one bout of 30 minutes of walking. Cardiovascular risk was reduced and mood was improved.

Myers J, Jullestad L, Vagelos R, et al. Clinical, hemodynamic and cardiopulmonary exercise test determinants of survival in patients referred for evaluation of heart failure. *Annals of Internal Medicine.* **1998 Aug 15; 129(4):286-293.**

644 people with at least 10 year history of heart failure were included in the study. Twelve factors were evaluated at base line. After 4 years, 187 patients (29%) died and 101 (16%) underwent heart transplantation. Researchers found that oxygen uptake (VO2) was the single most important factor in determining positive outcome in these patients.

Osterberg KKL and Melby CL. Effect of acute resistance exercise on postexercise oxygen consumption and resting metabolic rate in young women. *International Journal of Sport Nutrition and Exercise Meta-bolism.* **2000 Mar; 10(1):71-81.**

7 young women aged 22-36 were studied for post-exercise oxygen consumption, resting metabolic rate and resting fat oxidation. Researchers found that acute, strenuous resistance exercise is capable of producing modest, but prolonged elevations of post-exercise metabolic rate and possibly fat oxidation.

Sanchez-Quesada JL, Homs-Serradesanferm R, Serrat-Serrat J, et al. Increase of LDL susceptibility to oxidation occurring after intense, long duration aerobic exercise. *Atherosclerosis*. 1995 Dec; 118(2):297-305.

Six well-trained runners, previously fasted, ran continuously for 4 hours. Liquid and food intake was controlled during the experiment. Changes in LDL triglycerides was found to be associated with exercise rather than food-related. In other words, very intense exercise can have an unfavorable effect on lipoprotein metabolism.

Sesso HD, Pafafenbarger RS Jr and Lee IM. Physical activity and coronary heart disease in men: The Harvard Alumni Health Study. *Circulation*. 2000 Aug 29; 102(9):975-980.

12,510 men (age 39 to 88) were followed from 1977 through 1993. Physical activity was assessed at baseline and at multiple points during the 16 years. Total physical activity and vigorous activities showed the strongest reductions in CHD risk. The association between physical activity and a reduced risk of CHD also extended to men with multiple coronary risk factors.

Siegel AJ, Lewandrowski EL, Chun KY, et al. Changes in cardiac markers including B-natriuretic peptide in runners after the Boston Marathon. *American Journal of Cardiology*. 2001 Oct 15; 88(8): 920-923.

From 1996 to 2001 Boston Marathon runners provided blood samples before and after the race. Post-race results showed an imbalance in clotting and inflammatory factors known to set the stage for heart attack. Though none of the marathon runners suffered heart trouble during or after the marathon, researchers warn that high-risk individuals with high blood pressure, diabetes or other chronic conditions may want to avoid running in marathons.

Speed CA and Shapiro LM. Exercise prescription in cardiac disease. *The Lancet*. 2000 Oct 7; 356(9237):1208-1210.

Although the importance of physical activity to health has long been recognized, the prescription of exercise for patients with cardiac disease was popularized only in the 1960s, specifically in relation to coronary artery disease.

Williams PT, Stefanick MR, Vranizan KM and Wood PD. The effects of weight loss by exercise or by dieting on plasma high-density lipoprotein (HDL) levels in men with low, intermediate, and normal-to-high HDL at baseline. *Metabolism*. 1994 Jul; 43(7): 917-924.

130 men, aged 30 to 59, were randomized for 1 year to lose weight by exercise, by caloric restriction, or to make no effort to lose weight. Baseline HDL levels were documented. The increase in HDL cholesterol levels was significantly greater in the men who had low HDL at baseline.

Venkatraman JT, Leddy J, and Pendergast D.. Dietary fats and immune status in athletes: clinical implications. *Medicine and Science of Sports Exercise*, 2000 Jul; 32(7Suppl):S389-95.

Studies have shown that a low-fat, high carbohydrate diet (15% fat, 65% carbohydrates) typically eaten by athletes increases inflammatory and decreases immune factors, depresses anti-oxidants and negatively affects blood lipoprotein ratios. Increasing the dietary fat intake of athletes to 42% does not negatively affect immune competency or blood lipoproteins, whereas it improves endurance exercise performance for cyclists and runners.

Coenzyme Q10 for Heart Health

Bleske BE, Willis RA, Anthony M, et al. The effect of pravastatin and atorvastatin on coenzyme Q10. *American Heart Journal*. 2001 Aug; 142(2):E2.

Studies suggest that HMG-CoA reductive inhibitors reduce CoQ10 levels. 12 healthy volunteers received either 20mg pravastatin or 10mg atorvastatin for 4 weeks.

Burke BE, Neuenschwander R, and Olson RD. Randomized, double-blind, placebo-controlled trial of coenzyme Q10 in isolated systolic hypertension. *Southern Medical Journal.* 2001 Nov; 94(1):1112-1117.

83 adults with isolated systolic hypertension took 60mg of CoQ10 daily for 12 weeks. The mean reduction in systolic blood pressure was 17.8 mm HG. No patient exhibited orthostatic blood pressure changes. These results suggest that CoQ10 may be safely offered to hypertensive patients as an alternative treatment option.

Chopra RK, Goldman R, Sinatra ST, et al. Relative bioavailability of coenzyme Q10 formulations in human subjects. *International Journal of Vitamin and Nutrition Research.* 1998; 68(2):109-113.

The relative bioavailability of typically available forms of CoQ10 was compared with Q-Gel, a new soluble form on CoQ10. The Q-Gel was vastly superior to the typically available preparations. This means that lower doses of Q-Gel will be required to rapidly reach and maintain adequate blood CoQ10 values.

Folkers K, Drzewoski J, Richardson PC, et al. Bioenergetics in clinical medicine. XVI. Reduction of hypertension in patients by therapy with coenzyme Q10. *Research Communications in Chemical Pathology and Pharmacology.* 1981 Jan; 31(1):129-140.

Six untreated hypertensive patients and 10 treated patients still having elevated blood pressures took CoQ10. 87% showed reduction in systolic pressure; 68% showed reduction in diastolic pressure and 90% achieved reduction to normal blood pressure. Researchers conjectured that CoQ10 normalizes peripheral resistance rather than affecting cardiac regulation, and that the activity of CoQ10 results from an increase in levels of CoQ10 in vascular tissue.

Folkers K, Wolaniuk J, Simonsen R, et al. Biochemical rationale and the cardiac response of patients with muscle disease to therapy with coenzyme Q10. *Proceedings of the National Academy of Science,* 1985 Jul; 82(13):4513-4516.

Researchers studied 12 patients with muscular dystrophy and myopathy as well as impaired cardiac function. 8 received CoQ10 and 4 received placebo for 3 months. The results show that impaired myocardial function as well as skeletal muscle may be improved by CoQ10 therapy. CoQ10 is the only known substance that offers a safe and improved quality of life for patients have muscle disease, based on intrinsic bioenergetics.

Ghirlanda G, Oradei A, Manto A, et al. Evidence of plasma CoQ10-lowering effect of HMG-CoA reductase inhibitors: a double-blind, placebo-controlled study. *Journal of Clinical Pharmacology,* **1993 Mar; 33(3): 226-229.**
Researchers studied 10 healthy volunteers and 30 patients with high cholesterol who took statin drugs or placebo. Researchers studied pre- and post-lab results for 10 measures. CoQ10 was reduced by 40% after the treatment. CoQ10 is essential for the production of energy and has antioxidant properties. Reducing CoQ10 in the human body may cause membrane alteration and cellular damage.

Langsjoen H, Langsjoen P, Langsjoen P, et al. Usefulness of coenzyme Q10 in clinical cardiology: a long-term study. *Molecular Aspects of Medicine.* **1994; 15(S); 165-75.**
424 patients with 6 types of cardiovascular disease took CoQ10 in addition to their existing medical regimens. Within 18 months, 10 cardiac deaths (2.4%) occurred. 58% of the patients improved by one functional class and 28% improved by two classes. Overall medication requirements dropped. In conclusion, CoQ10 is a safe and effective adjunctive treatment for a broad range of cardiovascular diseases, producing positive clinical responses and easing the burden of multi-drug therapy.

Langsjoen P, Langsjoen P, Willis R and Folkers K. Treatment of essential hypertension with coenzyme Q10. *Molecular Aspects of Medicine.* **1994; 15 Suppl:S265-272.**
109 patients with hypertension were observed for several months after adding CoQ10 to their treatment. 51% of the patients discontinued 1 to 3 anti-hypertensive medications within 6 months; 91% of the patients showed significant improvement in both systolic and diastolic blood pressure.

Langsjoen PH, Langsjoen PH, and Folkers K. A six-year clinical study of therapy of cardiomyopathy with coenzyme Q10. International Journal of Tissue Reactivity. 1990; 12(3):169-171.

143 patients with cardiomyopathy were given 100mg of coenzyme Q10 in addition to conventional medical program in a 6 year study. Average CoQ10 levels rose from 0.85mcg to 2.0mcg in 3 months and stayed stable at that level. Mortality levels at 12 months and 24 months were much lower than would have been expects. Coenzyme Q10 is safe and effective long-term therapy for chronic cardiomyopathy.

Singh RB, Niaz MA, Rostogi SS, et al. Effect of hydrosoluble coenzyme Q10 on blood pressures and insulin resistance in hypertensive patients with coronary artery disease. Journal of Human Hypertension. 1999 Mar; 13(3):203-208.

59 patients using anti-hypertension medications were randomized into 2 groups, receiving either 120mg of CoQ10 or B vitamin complex for 8 weeks. The group taking CoQ10 experienced decreased blood pressure, blood insulin and glucose, triglycerides and lipids. CoQ10 improved HDL, vitamins A, C and E levels.

Yamagami T, Shibata N and Folkers K. Bioenergetics in clinical medicine. VIII. Administration of coenzyme Q10 to patients with essential hypertension. Research Communications in Chemical Pathology and Pharmacology. 1976 Aug; 14(4):721-727.

Coenzyme Q10 was administered to patients having essential hypertension for 3-5 months. Administration of the CoQ10 reduced both systolic and diastolic blood pressures, and increased the level of CoQ10 activity, presumably due to improved bioenergetics through correction of a deficiency of CoQ10.

Supplements for Heart Health

Auer W, Eiber A, Hostkorn E, et al. Hypertension and hyperlipi-daemia: Garlic helps in mild cases. *British Journal of Clini-cal Practical Supplements*. 1990 Aug; 69:3-6.

47 patients with mild hypertension took part in a trial where they either received garlic powder or a placebo for 12 weeks. Researchers monitored blood pressure and blood lipids at 4, 8, and 12 weeks. Sig-nificant differences were found. In the group taking garlic, their average diastolic (lower) blood pressure dropped from 102 to 89, and both cholesterol and triglycerides were significantly reduced. No significant changes occurred in the placebo group.

Barringer TA, Kirk JK, Santaniello AC, et al. Effect of a multivitamin and mineral supplement on infection and quality of life. A randomized, double-blind, placebo-controlled trial. *Annals of Internal Medicine.* **2003 Mar 4: 138(4):365-371.**

130 participants, aged 45-64, some with type 2 diabetes mellitus, took multivitamin and mineral supplement or placebo daily for 1 year. Participants receiving placebo reported more infectious illness than those taking the supplements (73% vs. 43%). 93% of diabetic patients on placebo reported infection, while only 17% of diabetic patients on supplements reported infection. Therefore, a multivitamin and mineral supplement reduced the incidence of infection, especially in the diabetic population.

Furman B, Rosenblat M, Hayek T, et al. Ginger extract consump-tion reduces plasma cholesterol, inhibits LDL oxidation and attenuates development of atherosclerosis in atherosclerotic apolipoprotein E-deficient mice. *Journal of Nutrition.* **2000 May; 130(5): 1124-1131.**

Researchers assumed that consumption of nutrients rich in antioxidants were associated with reduced development of atherosclerosis. Researchers worked with 60 mice divided into 3 groups – placebo, 25mcg ginger and 250mcg ginger. They found that adding ginger to the diet of the mice did, indeed, reduce the development of atherosclerosis and was associated with significant reduction in LDL cholesterol levels.

Graham IM, Daly LE, Refsum HM, et al. Plasma homocysteine as a risk factor for vascular disease: *The European Concerted Action Project. Journal of the American Medical Association.* **1997 June 22; 277(22):1775-1781.**

Nineteen centers in 9 European countries studied 750 people with vascular disease and 800 health people. An increased homocysteine level gave an independent risk of vascular disease similar to that of smoking or high cholesterol. When high homocysteine levels are combined with smoking or high cholesterol, the odds of vascular disease increased enormously. Researchers suggest doing studies of the effects of vitamins to reduce homocysteine levels and therefore vascular disease risk.

Guyton JR. Extended-release niacin for modifying the lipoprotein profile. *Expert Opinion on Pharmacotherapy.* **2004 June; 5(6):1385-1898.**

Niacin raises HDL, lowers triglycerides and LDL. One large trial monotherapy trial and multiple small trials of niacin in combination with lipid-modifying drugs show remarkable consistency in the ability of niacin to improve angiographic and clinical outcomes. Niacin extended-release represents an effective and safe option in the management of low levels of HDL and other lipoprotein abnormalities.

Kohlmeier L, Lark JD, Gomez-Gracia E, et al. Lycopene and myocardial infarction risk in the EURAMIC Study. *American Journal of Epidemiology.* **1997 Oct 15; 148(2):618-626.**

A multi-center study in 10 European countries studied people after they had heart attacks, looking for the presence of carotenes (related to Vitamin A). They concluded that lycopene seemed to provide a protective effect on heart attack risk.

Kurl S, et al. Plasma Vitamin C modifies the association between hypertension and risk of stroke. *Journal of the American Medical Association.* **2002 Sep 18; 288(11):1333.**

A 10-year study of 2,419 men (aged 42 to 60 at the beginning), found that 120 of the men had strokes. After examining 12 variables, they found that hypertension and obesity most increased the chances of a stroke. In addition, men with very low levels of Vitamin C had a 2.4-fold increased risk of stroke. Intake of Vitamin C is the easiest way to protect against the possibility of a stroke.

Mabile L, Bruckdorfer KR and Rice-Evans C. Moderate supplementation with natural alpha-tocopherol decreases platelet aggregation and low-density lipoprotein oxidation. *Atherosclerosis.* 1999 Nov 1; 147(1):177-185.

22 subjects took alpha-tocopheral (Vitamin E), 75 IU/day for 2 weeks, 200 IU/day for 2 weeks and 400 IU/day for 2 weeks. Results showed that uptake of vitamin E by platelets was optimal at 75 IU/day, correlating with the maximal influence on platelet aggregation and platelet responsiveness to inhibition by prostaglandin E.

Mottram P, Shige H, and Nestel P. Vitamin E improves arterial compliance in middle-aged men and women. *Atherosclerosis.* 1999 Aug; 145(2):399-404.

Loss of elasticity in large arteries is an emerging cardiovascular risk factor. Vitamin E may lower vascular resistance. 28 subjects were randomized to receive 8 weeks of 400 IU Vitamin E daily or a placebo. Arterial elasticity was increased 44% at 8 weeks in the Vitamin E group. No changes occurred in the placebo group.

Stampfer M, Malinow MR, Willett WC, et al. A prospective study of plasma homocyst(e)ine and risk of myocardial infarction in US physicians. *Journal of the American Medical Association.* 1992 Aug 19; 268(7):877-881.

14,916 men, aged 40 to 84, without prior heart attack or stroke, provided baseline blood samples and were followed for 5 years. 271 men subsequently developed heart attacks and were analyzed for homocystein levels. Moderately high levels of plasma homocystein are associated with subsequent risk of heart attack, independent of other risk factors. High levels of homocystein levels can be easily treated with vitamin supplements.

Stys T, Stys A, Kelly P and Lawson W. Trends in use of herbal and nutritional supplements in cardiovascular patients. *Clinical Cardiology.* 2004 Feb; 27(2):87-90.

The study sought to characterize cardiology patients who used supplements and to examine whether their use was diagnosis or doctor dependent, whether it affects patients' compliance, and what supplements were used. The use of supplements is widespread among cardiology patients. While it is not possible to predict which patients will use supplements, it appears that the use of supplements does not affect compliance with traditional medications.

Walker AF, Marakis G, Morris AP, and Robinson PA. Promising hypotensive effect of hawthorn extract: A randomized double-blind pilot study of mild, essential hypertension. *Phytotherapy Research,* 2002 Jan; 16(1):48-54.

36 patients with hypertension underwent baseline tests and then were assigned to daily supplements for 10 weeks of either (a) 600mg magnesium, (b) 500mg hawthorn extract, (c) both magnesium and hawthorn, or (d) placebo. Measurements at 65 and 10 weeks showed a decline in blood pressure in the groups taking hawthorn; these patients also reported a decrease in anxiety.

Wilburn AJ, King DS, Glisson J, et al. The natural treatment of hypertension. *Journal of Clinical Hypertension.* 2004 May; 6(5):242-248.

Researchers reviewed the efficacy of commonly available dietary supplements in the treatment of hypertension by measuring decrease in blood pressure. Supplements which lowered systolic blood pressure at least 9 mm Hg and/or diastolic blood pressure at least 5 mm Hg were coenzyme Q10, fish oil, garlic, vitamin C and L-arginine.

Wolf, RL, Cauley, JA, Baker, CE, et al. Factors associated with calcium absorption efficiency in pre- and perimenopausal women. *American Journal of Clinical Nutrition,* 2000 Aug; 72(2):466-471.

442 healthy pre- and perimenopausal women were studied for their absorption of calcium. The study showed that calcium absorption averaged 35%, with a range of 17-58%. Researchers found that lower dietary fat intake is significantly associated with lower calcium absorption values. Since calcium is already difficult for the body to absorb, anything that increases that difficulty is undesirable.

ABOUT THE AUTHOR

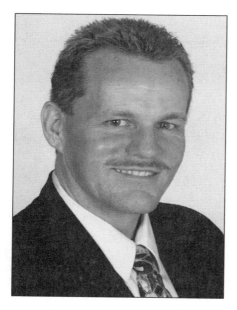

Dr. Al Sears owns and operates The Center for Health and Wellness, an integrative medicine and anti-aging clinic in south Florida, where he has treated more than 15,000 patients. Over the last 15 years, he has developed a revolutionary concept of integrative medicine by blending the best of modern Western medicine with the sciences of nutrition, herbal medicine, and exercise physiology. He founded The Wellness Research Foundation, a non-profit organization devoted to health research and education. His practice also includes the non-profit McCormick-Green Center for Integrative Therapies, the Library for Integrative Medicine, and an herbal apothecary of more than 250 organic herbs used for treatments, research, and education.

Dr. Sears has been appointed to the international panel of experts of the Health Sciences Institute, a worldwide information service for integrative healthcare. He is also an adjunct professor at Barry University, where he teaches courses in anatomy, human physiology, and nutrition. He is a member of the American Academy of Anti-Aging Medicine and is Board Certified in Anti-Aging Medicine.

Dr. Sears has written numerous articles and reports in the fields of natural health and nutritional supplementation. He writes the monthly publication *Health Confidential* and the twice weekly Internet Health Alerts. He has written the self-help prostate guide, *The 21st Century Men's Guide to Prostate Health* and *The T-Factor* book, which details nutritional and herbal strategies for increasing testosterone naturally.

Index

How to stay informed of the latest advances in diet and nutrition:

Visit **www.dragondoor.com/cgi-bin/tpost.pl** and participate in Dragon Door's stimulating and informative Diet and Nutrition Forum. Post your diet questions or comments and get quick feedback from leading nutrition experts.

Visit **www.dragondoor.com** and browse the Articles section and other pages for groundbreaking theories and products for improving your health and well being.

Call Dragon Door Publications at **1-800-899-5111** and request your FREE Vitalics catalog of fitness books, videos, supplements and equipment.

The Graduate Course In Instant Strength Gains

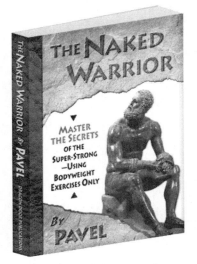

"Pavel has created a superb conditioning program with his newest book *"The Naked Warrior—Master the Secrets of the Super-Strong Using Bodyweight Exercises Only"*. It's a program of proven techniques to build a super strong body using simple bodyweight exercises. I truly believe that this is a great book for those who want to get in shape or stay in shape." – *Al Sears, M.D.*

The Naked Warrior
Master the Secrets of the Super-Strong—Using Bodyweight Exercises Only
By Pavel   #B28 $39.95
Paperback 218 pages 8.5" x 11"
Over 190 black & white photos plus illustrations

"If I was stuck on a desert island (or somewhere else with no access to weights) I'd hope that Pavel Tsatsouline would be there to help keep me in shape. With *The Naked Warrior*, Pavel has moved the art of exercise without weights to a new level. I like both the exercises he has selected and the approach he advocates for training on them. Now, whether you have weights or not, there is no reason not to get into top shape!"
—Arthur Drechsler, author *"The Weightlifting Encyclopedia"*

- **Gain** more brute strength in days than you did in years of bodybuilding or calisthenics
- **Discover** the martial secrets of instant power generation—for rapid surges in applied strength
- **Discover** how to get a world-class powerlifter's quality workout—using your body only
- **Get** a harder, firmer, functionally-fitter body—and be as resilient as hell whatever you face
- **Master** the one-arm/one-leg pushup for crushing upper body force
- **Forge** super-piston, never-quit legs with the Spetsnaz favorite "Pistol"
- **Discover** the magic of "GTG"—guaranteed the world's most effective strength routine
- **Be tow-truck strong**—yet possess the rugged looks of a stripped-down racer
- **No gym, no weights, no problem**—get a dynamite strength workout at a moment's notice—wherever you are

"Pavel's Naked Warrior DVD is worth its weight in gold!"

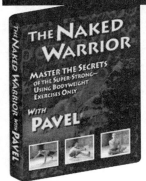

The Naked Warrior
Master the Secrets of the Super-Strong—Using Bodyweight Exercises Only with Pavel
DVD #DV015 $34.95

"As a diehard weightlifting competitor throughout the past 40 years, I at first viewed the bodyweight-only approach of *The Naked Warrior* with some trepidation. Imagine my surprise when discovering Pavel Tsatsouline's latest work stresses real STRENGTH TRAINING, employment of a limited amount of key major muscle group movements, and a high intensity, low rep format! Indeed, by deriving the best features of proven power building programs from all weightlifting disciplines, gymnastics, martial arts, and other "heavy" exercise modes, Mr. Tsatsouline has redefined strength-conditioning for the 21st century!"
—John McKean, six time All-Round Weightlifting World Champion

If you are looking for a
SUPREME EDGE
in your chosen sport
—seek no more!

Both the Soviet Special Forces and numerous world-champion Soviet Olympic athletes used the ancient Russian Kettlebells as their secret weapon for xtreme fitness. Thanks to the kettlebell's astonishing ability to turbocharge physical performance, these Soviet supermen creamed their opponents time-and-time again, with inhuman displays of raw power and explosive strength.

Now, former Spetznaz trainer, international fitness author and nationally-ranked kettlebell lifter, Pavel Tsatsouline, delivers this secret Soviet weapon into your own hands. You NEVER have to be second best again! Here is the first-ever complete kettlebell training program—for Western shock-attack athletes who refuse to be denied—and who'd rather be dead than number two.

PRAISE FOR *THE RUSSIAN KETTLEBELL CHALLENGE*

"In *The Russian Kettlebell Challenge*, Pavel Tsatsouline presents a masterful treatise on a superb old-time training tool and the unique exercises that yielded true strength and endurance to the rugged pioneers of the iron game. Proven infinitely more efficient than any fancy modern exercise apparatus, the kettlebell via Pavel's recommendations is adaptable to numerous high and low rep schemes to offer any strength athlete, bodybuilder, martial artist, or sports competitor a superior training regimen. As a former International General Secretary of the International All-Round Weightlifting Association, I not only urge all athletes to study Mr. Tsatsouline's book and try these wonderful all-round kettlebell movements, but plan to recommend that many kettlebell lifts again become part of our competitions!"—John McKean, current IAWA world and national middleweight champion

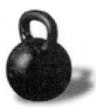

"Everybody with an interest in the serious matter of body regulation over a lifetime should commit themselves to Pavel's genre of knowledge and his distinct techniques of writing. Any one of the dozens of suggestions you hit upon will pay for the *Russian Kettlebell Challenge* hundreds of times."—Len Schwartz, author of *Heavyhands: the Ultimate Exercise System* and *The Heavyhands Walking Book!*

The Russian Kettlebell Challenge—

Xtreme Fitness for Hard Living Comrades

By Pavel Tsatsouline
Book #B15 $34.95
Paperback 170 pages

With Pavel Tsatsouline
Running Time: 32 minutes
DVD #DV001 $39.95

- **Get really, really nasty**—with a commando's wiry strength, the explosive agility of a tiger and the stamina of a world-class ironman
- **Own the single best conditioning tool** for killer sports like kickboxing, wrestling, and football
- **Watch in amazement** as high-rep kettlebells let you hack the fat off your meat—without the dishonor of aerobics and dieting
- **Kick your fighting system into warp speed**—with high-rep snatches and clean-and-jerks
- **Develop steel tendons and ligaments**—with a whiplash power to match
- **Effortlessly absorb ballistic shocks**—and laugh as you shrug off the hardest hits your opponent can muster
- **Go ape on your enemies**—with gorilla shoulders and tree-swinging traps

Look WAY YOUNGER than Your Age
Have a LEAN, GRACEFUL, Athletic-Looking Body
Feel AMAZING, Feel VIGOROUS, Feel BEAUTIFUL
Have MORE Energy and MORE Strength to
Get MORE Done in Your Day

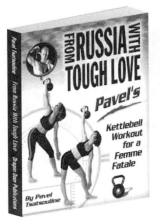

From Russia with Tough Love
Pavel's Kettlebell Workout for a Femme Fatale
Book #B22 $34.95 By Pavel Tsatsouline
Paperback 184 pages 8.5" x 11"

In Russia, kettlebells have long been revered as the fitness-tool of choice for Olympic athletes, elite special forces and martial artists. The kettlebell's ballistic movement challenges the body to achieve an unparalleled level of physical conditioning and overall strength.

But until now, the astonishing benefits of the Russian kettlebell have been unavailable to all but a few women. Kettlebells have mostly been the sacred preserve of the male professional athlete, the military and other hardcore types. That's about to change, as Russian fitness expert and best selling author PAVEL, delivers the first-ever kettlebell program for women.

It's wild, but women really CAN have it all when they access the magical power of Russian kettlebells. Pavel's uncompromising workouts give *across-the-board, simultaneous, spectacular and immediate results* for all aspects of physical fitness: strength, speed, endurance, fat-burning, you name it. Kettlebells deliver any and everything a woman could want—if she wants to be in the best-shape-ever of her life.

And one handy, super-simple tool—finally available in woman-friendly sizes—does it all. No bulky, expensive machines. No complicated gizmos. No time-devouring trips to the gym.

Into sports? Jump higher. Leap further. Kick faster. Hit harder. Throw harder. Run with newfound speed. Swim with greater power. Endure longer. Wow!

Working hard? Handle stress with ridiculous ease. Blaze thru tasks in half the time. Radiate confidence. Knock 'em dead with your energy and enthusiasm.

Can't keep up with your kids? Not any more! They won't know what hit them.

Just wanna have fun? Feel super-relaxed from the endorphin-rush of your life, dance all night and feel finer-than-fine the next morning...and the next...and the next.

Got attitude? Huh! Then try Pavel's patented Russian Kettlebell workouts. Now, THAT'S attitude!

Just some of what *From Russia with Tough Love* reveals:

- How the *Snatch* eliminates cellulite, firms your butt, and gives you the cardio-ride of a lifetime
- How to get as strong as you want, without bulking up
- How the *Swing* melts your fat and blasts your hips 'n thighs
- How to supercharge your heart and lungs without aerobics
- How to shrink your waist with the *Power Breathing Crunch*
- How the *Deck Squat* makes you super flexible
- An incredible exercise to tone your armsand shoulders
- The *Clean-and-Press*—for a magnificent upper body
- *The real secret to great muscle tone*
- The *Overhead Squat* for explosive leg strength
- How to *think* yourself stronger—yes, really!
- The queen of situps—for those who can hack it
- Cool combination exercises that deliver an unbelievable muscular and cardiovascular workout in zero time
- An unreal drill for a powerful and flexible waist, back, and hips
- How to perform multiple mini-sessions for fast-lane fitness

"Download this disc into your eager cells and watch in stunned disbelief as your body reconstitutes itself, almost overnight"

The Sure-Fire Secret to Looking Younger, Leaner and Stronger AND Having More Energy to Get a Whole Lot More Done in the Day

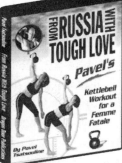

Spanking graphics, a kick-ass opening, smooth-as-silk camera work, Pavel at his absolute dynamic best, two awesome femme fatales, and a slew of fantastic KB exercises, many of which were not included on the original Russian Kettlebell Challenge video.

At one hour and twenty minutes of rock-solid, cutting-edge information, this video is value-beyond-belief. I challenge any woman worth her salt not to be able to completely transform herself physically with this one tape.

"In six weeks of kettlebell work, I lost an inch off my waist and dropped my heart rate 6 beats per minute, while staying the same weight. I was already working out when I started using kettlebells, so I'm not a novice. There are few ways to lose fat, gain muscle, and improve your cardio fitness all at the same time; I've never seen a better one than this."
—*Steven Justus, Westminster, CO*

"I have practiced Kettlebell training for a year and a half. I now have an anatomy chart back and have gotten MUCH stronger."
—*Samantha Mendelson,
Coral Gables, FL*

"Kettlebells are without a doubt the most effective strength/endurance conditioning tool out there. I wish I had known about them 15 years ago!"
—*Santiago, Orlando, FL*

"I know now that I will never walk into a gym again - who would? It is absolutely amazing how much individual accomplishment can be attained using a kettlebell. Simply fantastic. I would recommend it to anyone at any fitness level, in any sport.
—*William Hevener,
North Cape May, NJ*

"It is the most effective training tool I have ever used. I have increased both my speed and endurance, with extra power to boot. It wasn't even a priority, but I lost some bodyfat, which was nice. However, increased athletic performance was my main goal, and this is where the program really shines."
—*Tyler Hass, Walla Walla, WA*

From Russia with Tough Love

Pavel's Kettlebell Workout for a Femme Fatale
With Pavel Tsatsouline
Running Time: 1hr 12 minutes
DVD **#DV002 $29.95**

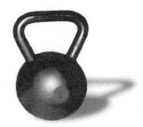

What you'll discover when "Tough" explodes on your monitor:

- The *Snatch*—to eliminate cellulite, firm your butt, and give you the cardio-workout of a lifetime
- The *Swing*— to fry your fat and slenderize hips 'n thighs
- The *Power Breathing Crunch*—to shrink your waist
- The *Deck Squat*—for strength and super-flexiblity
- The queen of situps—for a flat, flat stomach

- An incredible exercise to tone your arms and shoulders
- The *Clean-and-Press*—for a magnificent upper body
- The *Overhead Squat*—for explosive leg strength
- Combination exercises that wallop you with an unbelievable muscular and cardio workout

ANNOUNCING:

"The World's *Single Most Effective Tool* for Massive Gains in Strength, Speed and Athletic Endurance"

- Get thick, cable-like, hellaciously hard muscle
- Get frightening, whip-like speed
- Get stallion-like staying-power in any sport
- Get a, well, <u>god-like</u> physique
- Get the most brutal workout of your life, without having to leave your own living room
- Get way more energy in way less time
- Get a jack-rabbit's jumping power—and a jackhammer's strength
- Get it all—and then more, with Russian KB's

Discover why Russian Kettlebells are storming into "favored status" with US military, SWAT, NFL, MLB, powerlifters, weightlifters, martial artists—and elite athletes everywhere.

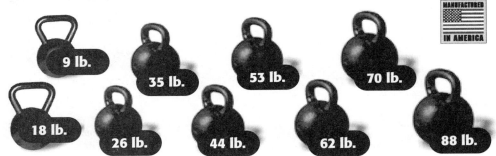

RUSSIAN KETTLEBELLS

STEEL HANDLE & CORE/RUBBER CASING		Price	MAIN USA	AK&HI	CAN
#P10D	4kg (approx. 9lb) —.25 poods	$89.95	S/H $10.00	$52.00	$29.00
#P10E	8kg (approx. 18lb) — .50 poods	$99.95	S/H $14.00	$70.00	$41.00

CLASSIC KETTLEBELLS (SOLID CAST IRON)

#P10G	12kg (approx. 26lb) — .75 poods	$82.95	S/H $20.00	$86.00	$53.00
#P10A	16kg (approx. 35lb) — 1 pood	$89.95	S/H $24.00	$95.00	$65.00
#P10H	20kg (approx. 44lb) — 1.25 poods	$99.95	S/H $28.00	$118.00	$72.00
#P10B	24kg (approx. 53lb) — 1.5 poods	$109.95	S/H $32.00	$137.00	$89.00
#P10J	28kg (approx. 62lb) — 1.75 poods	$129.95	S/H $36.00	$154.00	$102.00
#P10C	32kg (approx. 70lb) — 2 poods	$139.95	S/H $39.00	$173.00	$115.00
#P10F	40kg (approx. 88lb) — 2.5 poods	$179.95	S/H $52.00	$210.00	$139.00

SAVE! ORDER A SET OF CLASSIC KETTLEBELLS & SAVE $17.00

#SP10	Classic Set (one each of 16, 24 & 32kg)	$322.85	S/H $95.00	$405.00	$269.00

ALASKA/HAWAII KETTLEBELL ORDERING
Dragon Door now ships to all 50 states, including Alaska and Hawaii. We ship Kettlebells to Alaska and Hawaii via UPS 2nd Day Air service.

CANADIAN KETTLEBELL ORDERING
Dragon Door now accepts online, phone and mail orders for Kettlebells to Canada, using UPS Standard service. UPS Standard to Canada service is guaranteed, fully tracked ground delivery, available to every address in all of Canada's ten provinces. Delivery time can vary between 3 to 10 days.

IMPORTANT — International shipping quotes & orders do not include customs clearance, duties, taxes or other non-routine customs brokerage charges are the responsibility of the customer.

- KETTLEBELLS ARE SHIPPED VIA UPS GROUND SERVICE, UNLESS OTHERWISE REQUESTED.
- KETTLEBELLS RANGING IN SIZE FROM 4KG TO 24KG CAN BE SHIPPED TO P.O. BOXES OR MILITARY ADDDRESSES VIA THE U.S. POSTAL SERVICE, BUT WE REQUIRE PHYSICAL ADDDRESSES FOR UPS DELIVERIES FOR THE 32KG AND 40KG KETTLEBELLS.

REAL PEOPLE–REAL RESULTS
THE COMRADES SPEAK OUT

"I have been a training athlete for over 30 years. I played NCAA basketball in college, kick boxed as a pro for two years, made it to the NFL as a free agent in 1982, powerlifted through my 20's and do Olympic lifting now at 42. I have also coached swimming and strength athletes for over 20 years.I have never read a book more useful than **Power to the People!** I have seen my strength explode like I was in my 20's again—and my joints are no longer hurting."
—Carter Stamm, New Orleans, LA

"I have been following a regimen I got from *Power to the People!* for about seven weeks now. I have lost about 17lbs and have lost three inches in my waist. My deadlift has gone from a meager 180lbs to 255 lbs in that short time as well."
—Lawrence J. Kochert

"I learned a lot from Pavel's books and plan to use many of his ideas in my own workouts. *Power to the People!* is an eye-opener. It will give you new—and valuable—perspectives on strength training. You will find plenty of ideas here to make your training more productive."
—Clarence Bass, author of Ripped 1, 2 &3.

"A good book for the athlete looking for a routine that will increase strength without building muscle mass. Good source of variation for anyone who's tired of doing standard exercises."
—Jonathan Lawson, IronMan Magazine

"Like *Beyond Stretching* and *Beyond Crunches*, his other books, this is great. I think that it is the best book on effective strength training that I have ever read. This is not a book just about theory and principles. But Tsatsouline provides a detailed and complete outline of an exact program to do and how to customize it for yourself. It is very different from anything you have probably every read about strength training. The things he teaches in the book though won't just get you strong, if you want more than that, but can make you look really good—lean, ripped, and/or real big muscled if you want it. It's a very good book; the best available English-language print matter on the topic of strength training."
—Dan Paltzik

"This is a real source of no-b.s. information on how to build strength without adding bulk. I learned some new things which one can't find in books like *'Beyond Brawn'* or *'Dinosaur Training'*."
—Nikolai Pastouchenko, Tallahassee, Florida

"Forget all of the fancy rhetoric. If you are serious about improving your strength and your health buy this book and pay attention to what's provided. I started in January 2000 doing deadlifts with 200 lbs. Three months later I was at 365 lbs. Pavel knows what he is talking about and knows how to explain it simply. That's it."
—Alan, Indiana

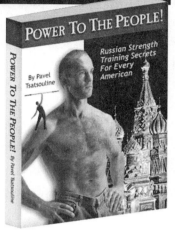

Power to the People!
Russian Strength Secrets for Every American **Book**
By Pavel Tsatsouline
Paperback 124 pages 8.5" x 11"
#B10 $34.95

"Brash and insightful, Power to the People is a valuable compilation of how-to strength training information. Pavel Tsatsouline offers a fresh and provocative perspective on resistance training, and charts a path to self-improvement that is both practical and elegantly simple. If building strength is your top priority, then *Power to the People* belongs at the top of your reading list."
—Rob Faigin, author of Natural Hormonal Enhancement

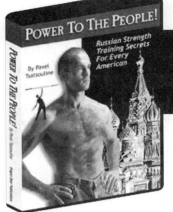
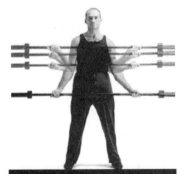

Be as FLEXIBLE as You Want to Be—FASTER, SAFER and SOONER

"I can't say I've read many books on flexibility with the wit and clear-headed wisdom I found in Pavel Tsatsouline's *Relax Into Stretch*. Tsatsouline delivers the how-and-why of progressive techniques for achieving suppleness, from simple yoga stretching to advance neuro-muscular facilitation, without burying the reader in hocus-pocus or scientific jargon. Tsatsouline's *Relax Into* Stretch provides an alternative: straightforward and practical techniques that don't require a lifetime to master".
—*Fernando Pages Ruiz, Contributing Editor Yoga Journal*

"I tell you truly that *Relax Into Stretch* is superb. Stretching has always been associated with any serious fitness effort and Tsatsouline's approach to this old discipline is fresh and unique and thought provoking. Best of all, this book combines philosophic insight with in-your-face reality as Pavel shares with the reader 'drills' that turn you into what this former Russian Spetznaz instructor calls ' a flexibility mutant'. This book supplies both the road map and the methodology. Don't ask to borrow my copy."
—*Marty Gallagher, Columnist, WashingtonPost.com*

"Pavel Tsatsouline's *Relax Into Stretch: Instant Flexibility Through Mastering Muscle Tension* is a superbly illustrated, step-by-step guide to achieve physical flexibility of muscle groups and sinews. *Relax Into Stretch* is very effective and very highly recommended reading for men and women of all ages and physical conditions seeking to enhance their mobility and flexibility as part of an overall exercise regimen."
—*Midwest Book Review*

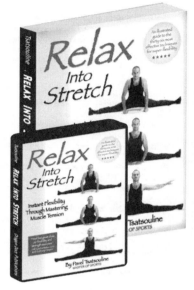

- Own an illustrated guide to the thirty-six most effective techniques for super-flexibility
- How the secret of mastering your emotions can **add immediate inches to your stretch**
- How to wait out your tension—the surprising key to greater mobility and a better stretch
- How to fool your reflexes into giving you all the stretch you want
- Why *contract-relax stretching* is 267% more effective than conventional relaxed stretching
- How to breathe your way to greater flexibility
- Using the Russian technique of *Forced Relaxation* as your **ultimate stretching weapon**
- How to stretch when injured—faster, safer ways to heal
- Young, old, male, female—learn what stretches are best for you and what stretches to avoid
- Why excessive flexibility can be detrimental to athletic performance—and how to determine your real flexibility needs
- Plateau-busting strategies for the chronically inflexible.

Here's what you'll discover, when you possess your own copy of Pavel Tsatsouline's *Relax Into Stretch:*

Stretching is NOT the best way to become flexible

Why Americans lose flexibility as they grow older • the dangers of physically stretching muscles and ligaments • *the role of antagonist passive insufficiency* • the nature and function of the *stretch reflex* • how to master muscular tension • how to inhibit the stretch reflex • intensive and extensive learning methods.

Waiting out the Tension— relaxed stretching as it should be

Just relax—when and when not to use the technique of *Waiting out the Tension* • Victor Popenko's key to mobility • the importance of visualization • why fear and anxiety reduce your flexibility • maximizing perceived safety in the stretch.

Proprioceptive Neuromuscular Facilitation

How Kabat's PNF fools your stretch reflex • the function of the *Renshaw cell* • why it works to pre-tense a stretched muscle.

Isometric stretching rules!

Why contract-relax stretching is 267% more effective than conventional relaxed stretching • what the 'frozen shoulder' has to teach us • the lifestyle problem of *'tight weakness'*, • why isometrics is more practical than weights.

Extreme flexibility through *Contrast Breathing*

How to breathe your way to greater flexibility • effective visualizations for the tension/release sequence • avoiding the dangers of hyperventilation.

Forced Relaxation—the Russian spirit of stretching

How to turn the contract-relax approach into a thermonuclear stretching weapon • determining correct duration • tips for the correct release of tension.

The final frontier: why *Clasp Knife* stretches will work when everything else fails

How to cancel out the *stretch reflex* • taking advantage of the *inverse stretch reflex* • the last line of defense against injuries • shutdown threshold isometrics • mastering the Golgi tendon reflex.

Why you should not stretch your ligaments— and how you can tell if you are

Yoga postures and stretches to avoid at all costs • the function and limitations of your ligaments.

Stretching when injured

Rest, Ice, Compression and Elevation • what happens when a muscle gets injured • contracting and releasing the injury • why stretching won't help a bad back and what to do instead.

The demographics of stretching

Why your age and sex should determine your stretches • the best—and worst—stretches for young girls, boys and adolescents • a warning for pregnant women • what's best for older folks.

The details, the schedule

Isometric stretches—when to do them and how often • how to know if you are doing too much • Bill 'Superfoot' Wallace's hardcore stretching schedule • correct order and choice of stretch • why isometric stretching should be the last exercise you do in your day.

The *Relax into Stretch* drills—

How much flexibility do you really need?

Why excessive flexibility can be detrimental to athletic performance • why old school strongmen instinctively avoided stretching • what stretches powerlifters and weightlifters do and don't need • warning examples from sprinting, boxing and kickboxing.

When flexibility is hard to come by, build strength

Plateau-busting strategies for the chronically inflexible • *high total time under tension.*

Two more plateau busting strategies from the iron world

Popenko's flexibility data • the reminiscence effect • the dynamic stereotype • How to exceed your old limits with the stepwise progression.

Advanced Russian Drills for Extreme Flexibility

Relax into Stretch delivers instant flexibility!

ORDERING INFORMATION

Customer Service Questions? Please call us between 9:00am– 11:00pm EST Monday to Friday at 1-800-899-5111. Local and foreign customers call 513-346-4160 for orders and customer service

100% One-Year Risk-Free Guarantee. If you are not completely satisfied with any product–for any reason, no matter how long after you received it–we'll be happy to give you a prompt exchange, credit, or refund, as you wish. Simply return your purchase to us, and please let us know why you were dissatisfied–it will help us to provide better products and services in the future. *Shipping and handling fees are non-refundable.*

Telephone Orders For faster service you may place your orders by calling Toll Free 24 hours a day, 7 days a week, 365 days per year. When you call, please have your credit card ready.

1·800·899·5111
24 HOURS A DAY
FAX YOUR ORDER (866) 280-7619

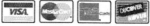

Complete and mail with full payment to: Dragon Door Publications, P.O. Box 1097, West Chester, OH 45071

Please print clearly

Sold To: A

Name_____

Street_____

City_____

State _____ Zip _____

Day phone*_____

* Important for clarifying questions on orders

Please print clearly

SHIP TO: *(Street address for delivery)* B

Name_____

Street_____

City_____

State _____ Zip _____

Email_____

Warning to foreign customers:
The Customs in your country may or may not tax or otherwise charge you an additional fee for goods you receive. Dragon Door Publications is charging you only for U.S. handling and international shipping. Dragon Door Publications is in no way responsible for any additional fees levied by Customs, the carrier or any other entity.

Warning!
This may be the last issue of the catalog you receive.

If we rented your name, or you haven't ordered in the last two years you may not hear from us again. If you wish to stay informed about products and services that can make a difference to your health and well-being, please indicate below.

Name_____

Address_____

City_____ State_____

Zip_____

ITEM #	QTY.	ITEM DESCRIPTION	ITEM PRICE	A OR B	TOTAL

HANDLING AND SHIPPING CHARGES • NO COD'S

Total Amount of Order Add:

$00.00 to $24.99	add	$5.00	$100.00 to $129.99	add $12.00
$25.00 to $39.99	add	$6.00	$130.00 to $169.99	add $14.00
$40.00 to $59.99	add	$7.00	$170.00 to $199.99	add $16.00
$60.00 to $99.99	add	$10.00	$200.00 to $299.99	add $18.00
			$300.00 and up	add $20.00

Canada & Mexico add $8.00. All other countries triple U.S. charges.

Total of Goods	
Shipping Charges	
Rush Charges	
Kettlebell Shipping Charges	
OH residents add 6% sales tax	
MN residents add 6.5% sales tax	
TOTAL ENCLOSED	

METHOD OF PAYMENT ___CHECK ___M.O. ___MASTERCARD ___VISA ___DISCOVER ___AMEX

Account No. *(Please indicate all the numbers on your credit card)*   EXPIRATION DATE

☐☐☐☐ ☐☐☐☐ ☐☐☐☐ ☐☐☐☐   ☐☐/☐☐

Day Phone (   )_____

SIGNATURE_____ DATE _____

NOTE: We ship best method available for your delivery address. Foreign orders are sent by air. Credit card or International M.O. only. For rush processing of your order, add an additional $10.00 per address. Available on money order & charge card orders only.

Errors and omissions excepted. Prices subject to change without notice.

City_____ State_____

Zip_____

Do You Have A Friend Who'd Like To Receive This Catalog?

We would be happy to send your friend a free copy. Make sure to print and complete in full:

Name_____

Address_____

City_____ State_____

Zip_____   DDP 11/04

ORDERING INFORMATION

Customer Service Questions? Please call us between 9:00am– 11:00pm EST Monday to Friday at 1-800-899-5111. Local and foreign customers call 513-346-4160 for orders and customer service

100% One-Year Risk-Free Guarantee. If you are not completely satisfied with any product–for any reason, no matter how long after you received it–we'll be happy to give you a prompt exchange, credit, or refund, as you wish. Simply return your purchase to us, and please let us know why you were dissatisfied–it will help us to provide better products and services in the future. *Shipping and handling fees are non-refundable.*

Telephone Orders For faster service you may place your orders by calling Toll Free 24 hours a day, 7 days a week, 365 days per year. When you call, please have your credit card ready.

1·800·899·5111
24 HOURS A DAY
FAX YOUR ORDER (866) 280-7619

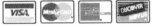

Complete and mail with full payment to: Dragon Door Publications, P.O. Box 1097, West Chester, OH 45071

Please print clearly

Sold To: A

Name_____

Street _____

City _____

State _____ Zip _____

Day phone*_____

* Important for clarifying questions on orders

Please print clearly

SHIP TO: *(Street address for delivery)*   B

Name_____

Street _____

City _____

State _____ Zip _____

Email _____

Warning to foreign customers:
The Customs in your country may or may not tax or otherwise charge you an additional fee for goods you receive. Dragon Door Publications is charging you only for U.S. handling and international shipping. Dragon Door Publications is in no way responsible for any additional fees levied by Customs, the carrier or any other entity.

Warning!
This may be the last issue of the catalog you receive.

If we rented your name, or you haven't ordered in the last two years you may not hear from us again. If you wish to stay informed about products and services that can make a difference to your health and well-being, please indicate below.

Name...

Address...

City .... State ....

Zip ....

Item #	Qty.	Item Description	Item Price	A or B	Total

HANDLING AND SHIPPING CHARGES • NO COD'S

Total Amount of Order Add:

$00.00 to $24.99	add $5.00	$100.00 to $129.99	add $12.00
$25.00 to $39.99	add $6.00	$130.00 to $169.99	add $14.00
$40.00 to $59.99	add $7.00	$170.00 to $199.99	add $16.00
$60.00 to $99.99	add $10.00	$200.00 to $299.99	add $18.00
		$300.00 and up	add $20.00

Canada & Mexico add $8.00. All other countries triple U.S. charges.

Total of Goods	
Shipping Charges	
Rush Charges	
Kettlebell Shipping Charges	
OH residents add 6% sales tax	
MN residents add 6.5% sales tax	
Total Enclosed	

METHOD OF PAYMENT ___CHECK ___M.O. ___MASTERCARD ___VISA ___DISCOVER ___AMEX

Account No. *(Please indicate all the numbers on your credit card)*   EXPIRATION DATE

☐☐☐☐ ☐☐☐☐ ☐☐☐☐ ☐☐☐☐   ☐☐/☐☐

Day Phone (   ) _____

SIGNATURE_____ DATE _____

NOTE: We ship best method available for your delivery address. Foreign orders are sent by air. Credit card or International M.O. only. For rush processing of your order, add an additional $10.00 per address. Available on money order & charge card orders only.

Errors and omissions excepted. Prices subject to change without notice.

Do You Have A Friend Who'd Like To Receive This Catalog?

We would be happy to send your friend a free copy. Make sure to print and complete in full:

Name ....

Address ....

City .... State ....

Zip .... DDP 11/04

ORDERING INFORMATION

Customer Service Questions? Please call us between 9:00am– 11:00pm EST Monday to Friday at 1-800-899-5111. Local and foreign customers call 513-346-4160 for orders and customer service

Telephone Orders For faster service you may place your orders by calling Toll Free 24 hours a day, 7 days a week, 365 days per year. When you call, please have your credit card ready.

100% One-Year Risk-Free Guarantee. If you are not completely satisfied with any product–for any reason, no matter how long after you received it–we'll be happy to give you a prompt exchange, credit, or refund, as you wish. Simply return your purchase to us, and please let us know why you were dissatisfied–it will help us to provide better products and services in the future. *Shipping and handling fees are non-refundable.*

1·800·899·5111
24 HOURS A DAY
FAX YOUR ORDER (866) 280-7619

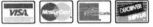

Complete and mail with full payment to: Dragon Door Publications, P.O. Box 1097, West Chester, OH 45071

Please print clearly

Sold To: A

Name_____

Street _____

City _____

State _____ Zip _____

Day phone*_____

* Important for clarifying questions on orders

Please print clearly

SHIP TO: *(Street address for delivery)* B

Name_____

Street _____

City _____

State _____ Zip _____

Email _____

Warning to foreign customers:
The Customs in your country may or may not tax or otherwise charge you an additional fee for goods you receive. Dragon Door Publications is charging you only for U.S. handling and international shipping. Dragon Door Publications is in no way responsible for any additional fees levied by Customs, the carrier or any other entity.

Warning!
This may be the last issue of the catalog you receive.

If we rented your name, or you haven't ordered in the last two years you may not hear from us again. If you wish to stay informed about products and services that can make a difference to your health and well-being, please indicate below.

Item #	Qty.	Item Description	Item Price	A or B	Total

Name_____

Address_____

City _____ State _____

Zip _____

HANDLING AND SHIPPING CHARGES • NO COD'S

Total Amount of Order Add:		
	$100.00 to $129.99	add $12.00
$00.00 to $24.99 add $5.00	$130.00 to $169.99	add $14.00
$25.00 to $39.99 add $6.00	$170.00 to $199.99	add $16.00
$40.00 to $59.99 add $7.00	$200.00 to $299.99	add $18.00
$60.00 to $99.99 add $10.00	$300.00 and up	add $20.00

Canada & Mexico add $8.00. All other countries triple U.S. charges.

Total of Goods	
Shipping Charges	
Rush Charges	
Kettlebell Shipping Charges	
OH residents add 6% sales tax	
MN residents add 6.5% sales tax	
TOTAL ENCLOSED	

Do You Have A Friend Who'd Like To Receive This Catalog?

We would be happy to send your friend a free copy. Make sure to print and complete in full:

METHOD OF PAYMENT ___CHECK ___M.O. ___MASTERCARD ___VISA ___DISCOVER ___AMEX

Account No. *(Please indicate all the numbers on your credit card)*   EXPIRATION DATE

☐☐☐☐ ☐☐☐☐ ☐☐☐☐ ☐☐☐☐   ☐☐/☐☐

Day Phone ( )_____

SIGNATURE_____ DATE _____

Name_____

Address_____

City _____ State _____

Zip _____

NOTE: We ship best method available for your delivery address. Foreign orders are sent by air. Credit card or International M.O. only. For rush processing of your order, add an additional $10.00 per address. Available on money order & charge card orders only.

Errors and omissions excepted. Prices subject to change without notice.

DDP 11/04

ORDERING INFORMATION

Customer Service Questions? Please call us between 9:00am– 11:00pm EST Monday to Friday at 1-800-899-5111. Local and foreign customers call 513-346-4160 for orders and customer service

100% One-Year Risk-Free Guarantee. If you are not completely satisfied with any product–for any reason, no matter how long after you received it–we'll be happy to give you a prompt exchange, credit, or refund, as you wish. Simply return your purchase to us, and please let us know why you were dissatisfied–it will help us to provide better products and services in the future. *Shipping and handling fees are non-refundable.*

Telephone Orders For faster service you may place your orders by calling Toll Free 24 hours a day, 7 days a week, 365 days per year. When you call, please have your credit card ready.

1·800·899·5111
24 HOURS A DAY
FAX YOUR ORDER (866) 280-7619

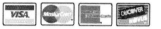

Complete and mail with full payment to: Dragon Door Publications, P.O. Box 1097, West Chester, OH 45071

Please print clearly

Sold To: **A**

Name_____

Street _____

City _____

State _____ Zip _____

Day phone*_____
Important for clarifying questions on orders

Please print clearly

SHIP TO: *(Street address for delivery)* **B**

Name_____

Street _____

City _____

State _____ Zip _____

Email _____

Warning to foreign customers:
The Customs in your country may or may not tax or otherwise charge you an additional fee for goods you receive. Dragon Door Publications is charging you only for U.S. handling and international shipping. Dragon Door Publications is in no way responsible for any additional fees levied by Customs, the carrier or any other entity.

Warning!
This may be the last issue of the catalog you receive.

If we rented your name, or you haven't ordered in the last two years you may not hear from us again. If you wish to stay informed about products and services that can make a difference to your health and well-being, please indicate below.

Item #	Qty.	Item Description	Item Price	A or B	Total

Name_____

Address_____

City _____ State _____

Zip _____

HANDLING AND SHIPPING CHARGES • NO COD'S

Total Amount of Order Add:

$100.00 to $129.99	add $12.00
$0.00 to $24.99 add $5.00	$130.00 to $169.99 add $14.00
$25.00 to $39.99 add $6.00	$170.00 to $199.99 add $16.00
$40.00 to $59.99 add $7.00	$200.00 to $299.99 add $18.00
$60.00 to $99.99 add $10.00	$300.00 and up add $20.00

Canada & Mexico add $8.00. All other countries triple U.S. charges.

Total of Goods	
Shipping Charges	
Rush Charges	
Kettlebell Shipping Charges	
OH residents add 6% sales tax	
MN residents add 6.5% sales tax	
Total Enclosed	

Do You Have A Friend Who'd Like To Receive This Catalog?

We would be happy to send your friend a free copy. Make sure to print and complete in full:

Name _____

Address _____

City _____ State _____

METHOD OF PAYMENT ___CHECK ___M.O. ___MASTERCARD ___VISA ___DISCOVER ___AMEX

Account No. *(Please indicate all the numbers on your credit card)* EXPIRATION DATE

▢▢▢▢ ▢▢▢▢ ▢▢▢▢ ▢▢▢▢   ▢▢/▢▢

Day Phone ( )_____

SIGNATURE_____ DATE _____

NOTE: We ship best method available for your delivery address. Foreign orders are sent by air. Credit card or International M.O. only. For rush processing of your order, add an additional $10.00 per address. Available on money order & charge card orders only.

Errors and omissions excepted. Prices subject to change without notice.

Zip _____

DDP 11/04

ORDERING INFORMATION

Customer Service Questions? Please call us between 9:00am– 11:00pm EST Monday to Friday at 1-800-899-5111. Local and foreign customers call 513-346-4160 for orders and customer service

100% One-Year Risk-Free Guarantee. If you are not completely satisfied with any product–for any reason, no matter how long after you received it–we'll be happy to give you a prompt exchange, credit, or refund, as you wish. Simply return your purchase to us, and please let us know why you were dissatisfied–it will help us to provide better products and services in the future. *Shipping and handling fees are non-refundable.*

Telephone Orders For faster service you may place your orders by calling Toll Free 24 hours a day, 7 days a week, 365 days per year. When you call, please have your credit card ready.

1·800·899·5111
24 HOURS A DAY
FAX YOUR ORDER (866) 280-7619

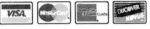

Complete and mail with full payment to: Dragon Door Publications, P.O. Box 1097, West Chester, OH 45071

Please print clearly

Sold To: A

Name_____

Street _____

City _____

State _____ Zip _____

Day phone*_____

* Important for clarifying questions on orders

Please print clearly

SHIP TO: *(Street address for delivery)*   B

Name_____

Street _____

City _____

State _____ Zip _____

Email _____

Warning to foreign customers:
The Customs in your country may or may not tax or otherwise charge you an additional fee for goods you receive. Dragon Door Publications is charging you only for U.S. handling and international shipping. Dragon Door Publications is in no way responsible for any additional fees levied by Customs, the carrier or any other entity.

Warning!
This may be the last issue of the catalog you receive.

If we rented your name, or you haven't ordered in the last two years you may not hear from us again. If you wish to stay informed about products and services that can make a difference to your health and well-being, please indicate below.

Name ....

Address ....

Item #	Qty.	Item Description	Item Price	A or B	Total

City .... State ....

Zip ....

HANDLING AND SHIPPING CHARGES · NO COD'S

Total Amount of Order Add:

$00.00 to $24.99 add $5.00	$100.00 to $129.99 add $12.00	
$25.00 to $39.99 add $6.00	$130.00 to $169.99 add $14.00	
$40.00 to $59.99 add $7.00	$170.00 to $199.99 add $16.00	
$60.00 to $99.99 add $10.00	$200.00 to $299.99 add $18.00	
	$300.00 and up add $20.00	

Canada & Mexico add $8.00. All other countries triple U.S. charges.

Total of Goods	
Shipping Charges	
Rush Charges	
Kettlebell Shipping Charges	
OH residents add 6% sales tax	
MN residents add 6.5% sales tax	
Total Enclosed	

Do You Have A Friend Who'd Like To Receive This Catalog?

We would be happy to send your friend a free copy. Make sure to print and complete in full:

METHOD OF PAYMENT ___CHECK ___M.O. ___MASTERCARD ___VISA ___DISCOVER ___AMEX

Account No. *(Please indicate all the numbers on your credit card)*   EXPIRATION DATE

☐☐☐☐ ☐☐☐☐ ☐☐☐☐ ☐☐☐☐   ☐☐/☐☐

Day Phone (   )_____

SIGNATURE_____ DATE _____

Name ....

Address ....

City .... State ....

NOTE: We ship best method available for your delivery address. Foreign orders are sent by air. Credit card or International M.O. only. For rush processing of your order, add an additional $10.00 per address. Available on money order & charge card orders only.

Errors and omissions excepted. Prices subject to change without notice.

Zip ....   DDP 11/04

ORDERING INFORMATION

Customer Service Questions? Please call us between 9:00am–11:00pm EST Monday to Friday at 1-800-899-5111. Local and foreign customers call 513-346-4160 for orders and customer service

100% One-Year Risk-Free Guarantee. If you are not completely satisfied with any product–for any reason, no matter how long after you received it–we'll be happy to give you a prompt exchange, credit, or refund, as you wish. Simply return your purchase to us, and please let us know why you were dissatisfied–it will help us to provide better products and services in the future. *Shipping and handling fees are non-refundable.*

Telephone Orders For faster service you may place your orders by calling Toll Free 24 hours a day, 7 days a week, 365 days per year. When you call, please have your credit card ready.

1·800·899·5111
24 HOURS A DAY
FAX YOUR ORDER (866) 280-7619

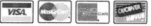

Complete and mail with full payment to: Dragon Door Publications, P.O. Box 1097, West Chester, OH 45071

Please print clearly

Sold To: **A**

Name_____

Street_____

City_____

State_____ Zip_____

Day phone*_____

Important for clarifying questions on orders

Please print clearly

SHIP TO: *(Street address for delivery)*   **B**

Name_____

Street_____

City_____

State_____ Zip_____

Email_____

ITEM #	QTY.	ITEM DESCRIPTION	ITEM PRICE	A OR B	TOTAL

Warning!
This may be the last issue of the catalog you receive.

If we rented your name, or you haven't ordered in the last two years you may not hear from us again. If you wish to stay informed about products and services that can make a difference to your health and well-being, please indicate below.

Name_____

Address_____

City_____ State_____

Zip_____

HANDLING AND SHIPPING CHARGES • NO COD'S

Total Amount of Order Add:		
$100.00 to $129.99	add	$12.00
$00.00 to $24.99 add $5.00	$130.00 to $169.99	add $14.00
$25.00 to $39.99 add $6.00	$170.00 to $199.99	add $16.00
$40.00 to $59.99 add $7.00	$200.00 to $299.99	add $18.00
$60.00 to $99.99 add $10.00	$300.00 and up	add $20.00

Canada & Mexico add $8.00. All other countries triple U.S. charges.

Total of Goods	
Shipping Charges	
Rush Charges	
Kettlebell Shipping Charges	
OH residents add 6% sales tax	
MN residents add 6.5% sales tax	
TOTAL ENCLOSED	

Do You Have A Friend Who'd Like To Receive This Catalog?

We would be happy to send your friend a free copy. Make sure to print and complete in full:

Name_____

Address_____

City_____ State_____

Zip_____

METHOD OF PAYMENT ___CHECK ___M.O. ___MASTERCARD ___VISA ___DISCOVER ___AMEX

Account No. *(Please indicate all the numbers on your credit card)*   EXPIRATION DATE

☐☐☐☐ ☐☐☐☐ ☐☐☐☐ ☐☐☐☐   ☐☐/☐☐

Day Phone (   )_____

SIGNATURE_____ DATE_____

NOTE: We ship best method available for your delivery address. Foreign orders are sent by air. Credit card or International M.O. only. For rush processing of your order, add an additional $10.00 per address. Available on money order & charge card orders only.

Errors and omissions excepted. Prices subject to change without notice.